Caroline's No Nightshade Kitchen Arthritis Diet

Living without Tomatoes, Peppers, Potatoes, and Eggplant

Caroline Thompson

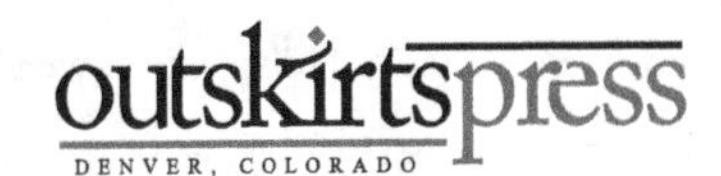

Caroline's No Nightshade Kitchen: Arthritis Diet
Living without tomatoes, peppers, potatoes, and eggplant!

v3.0

Outskirts Press, Inc.
http://www.outskirtspress.com

ISBN: 978-1-4327-9716-4

PRINTED IN THE UNITED STATES OF AMERICA

MYSTERIES OF NIGHTSHADES

Nightshades have a long history of use in medicine and cosmetics. Prior to the Middle Ages, the plants were used as an anesthetic for surgery; and ancient Romans used toxic nightshades as a poison. The wives of Emperor Augustus and Claudius both murdered contemporaries with these mysterious plants. Predating this time, nightshades were used to make poison arrows for battle.

Today, the relationship of nightshades and arthritis continues to be somewhat of a mystery to many in the medical profession. This may be due to the fact that nightshade toxins clearly do not affect everyone with arthritis, only some unknown percentage. However, those of us who regularly experience pain and joint swelling when we accidentally, or occasionally on purpose, ingest nightshade foods in any form, the results are authentic. Eating the forbidden tomato, potato, mild or hot pepper, and eggplant, causes a reaction that is painful and completely conclusive, over and over again. There is no mistaking the cause and effect.

Norman Childers, PhD, founder of the Arthritis Nightshades Research Foundation, conducted a study with over 1400 volunteers concerning this relationship. In his research paper, "An Apparent Relationship of Nightshades to Arthritis," published in 1993, in the *Journal of Neurological and Orthopedic Medical Surgery* (12:227-231), he concludes that "...nightshades are an important causative factor in arthritis in sensitive people." Additional information follows throughout this book, including many other sources and references in the appendix.

Hopefully future research, possibly gene identification, will provide conclusive scientific results that will enable those with arthritis to determine if nightshade plants are causing, or adding to, their crippling affliction. The Center for Disease Control reports that over twenty-one million people are affected, and often disabled, with arthritis in this country. The numbers are staggering. If you suffer from arthritis, why not do what I did. Stop ingesting nightshades for a few weeks and see for yourself.

Caroline Thompson

IN APPRECIATION

This book is dedicated to my husband
George Thompson
with gratitude for his loving support
beyond my wildest dreams

Special Thanks
for editing,
testing recipes, sharing recipes,
and amazing support
Mary Kay Stoehr, Cassie Armstrong,
Carol Grever, Valerie Sterling, Jeanne Baughman, Virginia Gridley,
Pat Wright, Peggy Mansfield, Dasha Durian,
Diana Wilson, Marysia Mycielski, Bo and Cynthia Stephens,
Coila Maphis, Susan Eriksson. Claire Jones Kneer,
Kelli Thompson Ivy, Andrew Jones, Holli Thompson Tomme,
Susan Henry Clark, Niki Hayden, Nan Fogel, Julie Mock,
Kathy Abernathy, Cathy Sanford, Martha Peacock,
and Patrice Morrow

Special thanks also to the many friends who believed in this project, who gave unending encouragement, and who helped make this cookbook a reality.

TABLE OF CONTENTS

CAROLINE'S NO NIGHTSHADE KITCHEN: ARTHRITIS DIET

A unique and unusual cookbook

Caroline Thompson

Welcome to ***Caroline's No Nightshade Kitchen: Arthritis Diet.*** It has been a joy creating this cookbook and recipes. My primary motivation has been to share what I've learned about nightshades and the harm this plant family causes many of those suffering from the symptoms of arthritis, rheumatoid arthritis, multiple sclerosis, gout, and other inflammatory illnesses. In the process, I've learned that many who have an extreme sensitivity to nightshades may have adverse reactions to gluten and lactose, which can also promote inflammation. Many of the recipes in my cookbook are gluten and lactose free.

When I first discovered the impact of nightshades on my body and in particular my hands, I was overcome by disappointment. I loved tomatoes, peppers, white potatoes, and eggplant. They were in most of my food selections, as they are for many of us. The prospective changes in my diet were overwhelming, and I didn't know where to begin. To be honest, it took effort and commitment to avoid nightshades at first, but avoiding them slowly became the norm for me. As this happened, I began to feel differently about my arthritis and the foods I had given up. I felt better physically, my attitude was brighter, and my commitment was strengthened by the progress I was making with the inflammation in my hands. My food plan became an adventure, and the responses of my family and friends were encouraging because I realized I was not the only one enjoying these new recipes. Without reservation, it became apparent to me that I needed to tell my story about my experiences with arthritis and write this cookbook.

Caroline's No Nightshade Kitchen: Arthritis Diet is an important book, and I hope you will read it and take what I have to say seriously. The history surrounding nightshades and their effect on arthritis, and possibly other types of pain, has been around for centuries, but it was often dismissed as folklore. However, like so many others, I experienced this folklore first hand and became a believer. My sensitivity to nightshades increased over the years, and it only took a few bites of nightshade foods, or seasonings, for me to have a severe reaction. You can understand why I'm serious about nightshades. Arthritis changed my life, and now I'm changing it again with a diet that gives me freedom from pain.

There's much more to explain about nightshades in the chapters ahead. I hope what I've experienced and learned about nightshades, arthritis, and inflammation will be a help to you. I also hope you will enjoy my recipes as much as I have enjoyed creating them and writing this book.

Nevertheless, let me begin my story and explain how I discovered the dangers of nightshade plants fourteen years ago.

My simple story and fourteen year history

In 1998, I began to notice pain, redness, and swelling in the knuckles of my hands. The pain was sudden and had never happened before. The discomfort in my hands became severe. I couldn't sleep, and I walked around with my hands elevated, hoping that would help ease the pain. I'm an abstract oil painter and need my hands to create art, and I was concerned that I would lose my ability to paint. It became apparent that not only would I be unable to paint, but there were other things I could no longer do well. Simple movements needed for housekeeping, gardening, and cooking caused me pain. Often I was unable to begin, or even complete, these ordinary tasks. Holding a book to read for any length of time became unbearable. I was frightened and there seemed to be no end to the misery. It never occurred to me that the inflammation I was experiencing in my hands could be related to the hot chili peppers and tomatoes I ate almost every day.

During the next three years, I went to many doctors who administered every arthritis prescription available at the time, but the medications actually made the pain and swelling worse. As the pain intensified, my discouragement became overwhelming. An orthopedic surgeon put my hands in casts, hoping to improve the structure of my bones and reduce the pain. The pressure of the casts against my hands and swollen knuckles was unbearable. The orthopedic surgeon also injected cortisone into the joints of my hands, which was excruciating and didn't help. I was sent to a rheumatologist who tested me for every strain of arthritis on record, but he could only say my particular type of arthritis was definitely an inflammatory reaction, but it was not found on traditional arthritis registries. I spent thousands of dollars trying to find an answer that would give me relief, but my discomfort only increased. I felt hopeless and desperate as the pain intensified and the disfiguration of my hands worsened.

One of my physicians gave me a genetic test to see if I had the arthritis gene. He was hoping to find a clue that might provide some answers. The results of the genetic test showed that I did have the gene, but not the classic arthritis gene. The report I received said that I had a genetic proclivity for arthritis inflammatory reactions, and I could see and feel the results. As before, the diagnosis I received was confusing but not helpful. Medical science had failed to answer my questions.

In 2001, I was visiting a friend who has a medical background and is knowledgeable about numerous types of alternative healthcare. She noticed my bright red, swollen hands and asked if I knew anything about nightshade plants and arthritis. She explained that the nightshade family of plants (tomatoes, peppers, white potatoes, and eggplant) had been proven to affect some people severely who have arthritis. I thought she was crazy. I couldn't believe giving up many of the foods I enjoyed eating could or would make a difference for me.

However, because the pain had been so severe for three years, and I was truly desperate for relief, she convinced me to change my diet for four weeks to see what might happen. Giving up tomatoes, peppers, white potatoes, and eggplant was a serious endeavor for me, because these four food categories were the mainstay in most of my cooking. I loved to cook and I especially loved tomatoes, peppers, and hot spices.

As I looked at my daily diet, I found that all three of my meals were especially prominent in tomatoes and peppers, the spicier the better. I could eat jalapenos and Thai chili paste with the best of them, and I often did. Could I live without these amazing flavors? Could I maintain a food plan that would limit these choices? I wasn't sure, but I was desperate and didn't have anything to lose, except a little time without nightshades.

I began the experiment my friend suggested the next day, but I had little hope a diet without nightshades would lessen my pain. I had been encouraged by the medical community before and expected more disappointment. The test to determine if you have sensitivity to nightshades is outlined in the **Basics about nightshades and their effect on arthritis**, which will be discussed later in this chapter.

I try to refrain from using the word miracle; but to be honest it was a miracle to me because the pain, redness, and swelling stopped completely in a few days. For some, it can take up to four weeks to see relief, or for their bodies to flush the toxin build up from nightshades. There is also data that states it can take up to six months for some individuals to flush the toxins completely from their systems. I was fortunate that improvement came quickly, and I'm grateful that my friend spoke up when she did.

Foolishly, after several years of living pain free, I began to gravitate back to nightshades. I wanted to try tomatoes and peppers again. At this point, after being completely free from nightshade toxins for several years, I found that I could eat tomatoes and peppers in small amounts on occasion, and although I would experience discomfort almost immediately, the pain, swelling, and redness would only last a couple of hours. I didn't eat nightshades often, but every time I did, I had the same results. The onset of pain would begin in thirty minutes to one hour after eating nightshades, last a couple hours, and then go away. Regrettably, I thought I could enjoy a few savory, small bites of nightshades without doing additional damage to the joints in my hands. Little did I realize that I was building an even more intense intolerance to nightshades. I had no idea what was haunting me or what would follow. Could the disfiguration of my hands, which increased during this time, have been avoided if I'd not played around with nightshades?

I've talked with people who say they realize that they've had sensitivity to nightshade foods for many years, have experienced pain and inflammation when they ate these foods, but chose not give up them up. Some people tell me they only have disfiguration from arthritis, without pain, so nightshades don't affect them. Others have said that their doctors tell them that arthritis in their knees or hips will cause them to have joint replacement surgery at some point. I wonder how many more people could be helped by the elimination of nightshade plants from their diets. Is this a larger problem than was first thought? Is damage occurring even when there is no apparent pain?

In the summer of 2010, a season abundant with all kinds of fresh, luscious vegetables, especially tomatoes and peppers, I noticed the level of pain and swelling in my hands had intensified and would not go away. Once again, it became as severe as in my earlier days with arthritis. I wanted to believe that I could flirt with nightshades, getting by with minor discomfort on occasion, but I was wrong. By summer's end, I had to face the fact that my sensitivity to nightshade plants had taken hold of my body, but this time it affected my body with a vengeance. Finally, with full resolve and commitment to abstain from all forms of nightshade plants, raw, cooked, or in spice form, I was again pain free.

Just as before, by maintaining this abstinence from nightshades, the pain, inflammation, and swelling subsided quickly and stayed away. The disfiguration in my hands didn't improve and probably never will, but I can live a life free of pain. Unfortunately, the damage has weakened my grip, which has been compromised by the inflammation.

Like many other health related issues, I believe allergies, sensitivities, or reactions to specific toxins can run in families. My father, who was born with a deformity in his feet and ankles, also suffered from a type of arthritis that his doctors could never pinpoint. His diagnosis was vague, just as mine would be years later. The treatments and medications he was given did little to help eliminate his pain, which was often severe to the point that he couldn't walk. My father loved to cook, and he especially loved spicy foods and peppers. Like father, like daughter, we both craved hot foods. He died many years ago, but what if eliminating nightshades from his diet could have made a difference for him? He suffered more than I can say with arthritis in his ankles, with little or no relief. Nothing would have made me happier than to ease the agony he endured for so long.

If you suffer from arthritis, I hope you'll try eliminating nightshades from your diet for four weeks, using the test I describe in detail later. As I said earlier, relief may come sooner, but please be patient and give it time. It's worth the effort, and your health and well-being might significantly improve. This phenomenon probably doesn't affect all types of arthritis, but if it affects you and you discover relief from joint pain and inflammation, I'll be extremely happy and so will you.

I'm not a medical professional and I don't have all the answers. I wish it were as simple as taking a pill, but it's not. I only know what I've experienced over the past fourteen years and what others have experienced and shared with me. As I've said many times, this strange but simple dietary elimination doesn't affect everyone, and I don't know why. Arthritis is a mysterious, crippling, cruel disease that has baffled science all through the ages. However, I do believe nightshades are a factor for many people, causing serious pain and suffering for them as they do for me.

Caroline's No Nightshade Kitchen: Arthritis Diet is my story with nightshades. It's also my personal collection of easy to follow recipes, which provide savory food options for you to enjoy. There is no reason to give up delicious dining experiences. I love to entertain and doubt if my guests miss the tomatoes, peppers, white potatoes, and eggplant that are no longer included in the plans for my meal.

Changing your diet to remove toxic nightshade foods is as easy as making a few changes in the foods you eat. In the next several chapters, you'll discover ways to replace nightshades with choices that are truly satisfying. Once you begin developing this new food plan, these simple changes will become second nature, and you'll experience a menu rich in luscious alternatives. Cooking and dining are opportunities for pleasure, and they should not make you sick.

May your good health be enhanced by your new adventures in cooking and dining.

Basics about nightshades and their effect on arthritis

The Center for Disease Control reports that arthritis is the most common cause of disability in the United States, limiting the activities of nearly twenty-one million adults. Many factors seem to cause arthritis pain, swelling, and sometimes disfiguration and crippling. There are numerous remedies, prescriptions, and theories regarding relief. Eliminating nightshades from the diet seems to help many, and it's the reason I have written this book. If you find that nightshades affect you, you may experience relief by avoiding these foods. The relief from nightshades that I discovered over many years changed my life.

Nightshades are a diverse group of foods, herbs, shrubs, and trees that have fascinated scientists, doctors, and nutritionists for centuries. Nightshade is actually the common name used to describe over 2,800 species of plants, many with different properties. This diverse category even includes plants such as tobacco and morning glory.

Numerous websites on the Internet explain the theory about the impact of nightshades on arthritis. One website of notable interest is by Norman F. Childers, PhD, who founded the Arthritis Nightshades Foundation in 1996. Dr. Childers concludes in his article, "An Apparent Relation of Nightshades to Arthritis," (*Journal of Neurological and Orthopedic Medical Surgery*, 1993) 12:227-231, "Diet appears to be a factor in the etiology of arthritis based on surveys of over 1400 volunteers during a 20-year period. Plants in the drug family, *Solanaceae* (nightshades) are an important causative factor in arthritis in sensitive people. This family includes potato (*Solanum tuberosum* L.), tomato (*Lycopersicon esculentum* L.), eggplant (*Solanum melongena* L.), tobacco (*Nicotiana tabacum* L.), and peppers (*Capsicum* sp.) of all kinds, except black pepper (family, *Piperaceae*). Rigid omission of *Solanaceae*, with other minor diet adjustments, has resulted in positive to marked improvement in arthritis and general health."

Because arthritis affects millions of people in the U.S., the sensitivity to nightshade plants may be more common than first thought. The level of pain caused by inflammation in the joints has varying degrees of severity for those suffering from it. The pain sometimes increases without the person knowing or understanding what is happening to him or her. Could dietary factors be affecting the joints and contribute to the increased discomfort? Arthritis research on the many facets of the disease is continuing. The disease is complex and has numerous issues and physical complications. How the disease physically affects each person with arthritis varies. The age of onset for the disease is unpredictable, because it affects both children and seniors. The treatment that provides relief for one individual may differ significantly for someone else. The thread connecting the disease is vague.

Because nightshade foods are prevalent in most American diets, these foods are difficult to avoid. Potatoes, tomatoes, sweet and hot peppers of all kinds, eggplant, paprika, cayenne, and bottled hot sauces are found in numerous commercially produced foods and in recipes that have been treasured and passed down in families for generations.

Lesser-known nightshade examples include ground cherries, tomatillos, garden huckleberry, and pimentos. Therefore, pimento cheese and pimento stuffed olives are examples of foods that may cause severe pain for certain individuals with arthritis. Although sweet potato is a distant relative of the nightshades, it does not belong to the plant family *Solanaceae,* which can affect arthritic joints. In addition, most individuals with arthritis can safely eat black and white peppers, other distant nightshade relatives. Although from the same plant, black pepper is picked while green and then dried in the sun until black. White pepper develops completely on the vine. Sweet potato, as well as black and white peppers, provides good alternatives in many of the recipes that appear in this book.

A particular group of substances in the nightshade plant family called alkaloids can react with the immune system in some people, which may affect nerve, muscle, and joint function. Because the amount of alkaloids is very low in nightshade foods, it is believed that only individuals with an extremely high sensitivity to this chemical are affected by the nightshade group. However, for the individuals in this group, alkaloids can cause extreme inflammation and sometimes pain.

Not everyone who has arthritis symptoms and disfiguration experiences extreme discomfort. The phenomenon of this toxic reaction seems isolated to a group of people who have established a high sensitivity to nightshades, probably over many years. While cooking nightshades lowers alkaloid content by about forty-fifty percent, the cooking process does not reduce the reaction in people who are highly sensitive to these foods. This sensitivity may be analogous to bee and wasp stings, which become more toxic as a person is repeatedly stung. As with multiple stings, the sensitivity buildup from nightshade toxicity becomes more intense over time with increased exposure to these foods. On a personal note, when I first discovered that nightshades significantly affected the pain I was experiencing, I noticed that I had very little effect from white potatoes and eggplant. Today, however, both white potatoes and eggplant, even in small amounts, cause me extreme pain, just as tomatoes and peppers do. I attribute this to an increased buildup in sensitivity to nightshades over the past fourteen years.

Just as people buildup sensitivity to nightshades, the plants need to evolve to protect themselves. As a result, nightshade plants have developed a means of defending themselves against predator insects that wish to eat them. The evolution of these plants has produced a toxic substance, or alkaloids, that protect them. Unfortunately, this same toxic barrier, which is important to the species' protection, apparently causes many people with arthritis to suffer pain and discomfort. Alkaloids seem to be the link that ties the nightshade plants together.

Nightshades have been used in pharmaceuticals since ancient times. Commonly known drugs, such as mandrake, belladonna, and bittersweet nightshade, were developed from certain nightshade plants. In legend, deadly nightshade (or belladonna), is said to belong to the devil who tends it in his leisure and is only diverted from his care one night each year, which is on Walpurgis, the witches' Sabbath.

Over the centuries, nightshades, and the beliefs surrounding them, have existed throughout folklore. In his book, *The History of Scotland*, George Buchanan, author, scholar, and historian (1506-1582), relates a tale of Macbeth poisoning the Danes, an invading army, with liquor contaminated with deadly nightshade. He offered the drink to the Danes during a truce. The invaders drank heavily, became easy prey, and were murdered in their sleep by the Scots.

Centuries ago, Italian women used small amounts of juice from deadly nightshade to dilate the pupils of their eyes, which was a sign of beauty. Scopolamine was added to morphine in1902, which caused a "twilight sleep" that lessened the pain and mortality of childbirth. This chemical was also used as a "truth serum" in many legal battles and court cases, which is still used in some countries today. Legends say that witches used a mixture of belladonna, opium poppy, and other poisonous plants to create "flying ointments," which they supposedly used when flying to other witch gatherings. In reality, these ointments encouraged hallucinatory dreams.

Seasonings and flavor additives can be a problem for the person who needs to avoid nightshades. Many commercially processed foods that are popular today contain paprika, cayenne, bell pepper, and other nightshades. These ingredients may be insignificant on the ingredients label but can do serious, permanent damage in terms of joint distortion and cripple those of us who have developed a high degree of sensitivity to nightshades.

As mentioned earlier, it is helpful to note that black or white peppers are not members of the *Solanaceae* family and do not cause harm for most people. These seasonings, along with dry mustard, horseradish, and wasabi, are additives that can safely provide spicy heat to many dishes. Specialty spice shops are excellent sources for other hot seasonings that can be used to replace the heat once enjoyed from nightshades. Curry powders are also available that do not contain cayenne and paprika. Fresh, minced ginger, and especially Thai ginger, can spice up many foods.

Potato starch, which should be avoided by those who are sensitive to nightshades, is found in many processed or prepared foods at the grocery store. This product is an additive in many canned soups, meats, etc. Some Worcestershire sauces contain chili extract and those sensitive to nightshades should avoid their consumption. It is important on many levels to read the ingredients label carefully on processed foods. (Please see: *Beverages, Sauces, and Other Fun Stuff,* for an alternative recipe for Worcestershire sauce.)

Eating in restaurants can be challenging. When dining out, it's important to ask the waiter questions about the ingredients in your food. When you mention that you have an "allergy" to certain foods, restaurant staffs are usually very helpful. However, even if the particular dish you order has no apparent nightshades in it, you may discover secret ingredients in sauces that will cause pain, such as potato starch, paprika, or cayenne. Unfortunately, a small amount of these seasonings can cause severe results for those with a high sensitivity to the plant family, *Solanaceae.*

Not only individuals with various forms of arthritis, but those experiencing joint problems such as gout and other inflammatory illnesses, may find physical relief by eliminating nightshades from their diets. For example, some individuals with multiple sclerosis have benefited from avoiding nightshades. Since these inflammatory diseases can attack different parts of the body, it's important to be aware of any isolated body areas that may experience pain, inflammation, or swelling.

Many researchers believe that there is an inflammatory correlation between nightshade plants, gluten foods, and lactose products. Some individuals, who have experienced arthritis relief by eliminating nightshades from their diets, are finding improved results by eliminating gluten and lactose as well. In this cookbook, all recipes are nightshade free, but where noted, recipes will also be gluten and/or lactose free.

It has been said that seventy-five percent of all people have an adverse reaction to one or more foods they consume. Symptoms vary but may include difficulty breathing, cough, fatigue, headache or migraine, flushing, rashes, swelling, and gastrointestinal difficulties (including gas, diarrhea, bloating, nausea, or abdominal pain). Peanut and shellfish allergies can be extremely life threatening. All sensitivities to food products and food items should be taken seriously. If you have concerns about a possible situation with any food you consume, please check with your medical professional or nutritional advisor.

Test for determining sensitivity to nightshades

1. As a test, eliminate all nightshade foods, including tomatoes, mild to hot peppers in all forms, white potatoes of all types, and eggplant from your diet. This also includes potato starch, bottled hot sauces, and relishes, such as spicy oriental pastes, ground paprika, and cayenne.

2. Allow up to four weeks for any existing toxicity to flush from your system. Relief may come more quickly for some, but please allow ample time for this to happen. If you have this sensitivity, remember that the smallest amount of nightshades in your system can cause an extreme reaction. The onset of pain and swelling can occur anywhere between thirty minutes to a few hours after consumption.

3. When you are completely pain and inflammation free, you may choose to test each category of the nightshades individually to determine if all forms of these plants trigger discomfort. Some individuals have a sensitivity to only one or two types of nightshades (especially in the early stages of sensitivity), although that sensitivity may be extreme. It's important to test each nightshade category individually.

4. If you become pain free after eliminating nightshades and determine that you're sensitive to this plant family, it will be necessary to be diligent about reading ingredient labels on processed foods, asking questions in restaurants about ingredients, and being aware of everything you're eating. If you have the sensitivity to nightshades, remember even a small amount can trigger severe pain, possibly followed by permanent disfiguration or crippling.

Let's begin

You are about to discover an approach to eating and cooking that has helped numerous individuals with arthritis live pain free. Many will say, "I've eaten these foods all my life, so why would nightshades harm me now and not harm everyone with arthritis?" Well, the answer may be simple. Over the years, certain people with this high sensitivity can experience an increased reaction to the alkaloids found in the plant family *Solanaceae*. As stated earlier, the physical occurrence of alkaloids in the body may respond with severe pain or other adverse reactions. For centuries, nightshades have been associated with pain, but this was often dismissed as folklore. In recent years, researchers found that there is a positive correlation between these plants and physical pain and inflammation.

If you suffer from nightshade sensitivity, this cookbook is designed for you. You can live relatively pain free without losing the enjoyment of eating delicious foods. In the following chapters, you'll find alternatives to cooking without nightshades by using these tested recipes, some complex and some very simple. These recipes will help satisfy your cravings for the foods you once enjoyed but will also delight your friends and family. My recipes are especially for you, but they are also for anyone who enjoys good food and loves to cook. In reality, eliminating nightshades from your diet is a small lifestyle change compared to the benefits you may receive to your health and well-being. There's not much to lose, and there are many delicious foods to savor along the way.

When I began this cookbook, my goal was to educate people suffering from arthritis pain about nightshades and to share what I found to be beneficial for many of us. It appears that many more individuals suffer from nightshade sensitivities than I first thought. These people include not only those with osteoarthritis but many suffering from rheumatoid arthritis, multiple sclerosis, and gout also share this sensitivity. Young and old, these diseases attack relentlessly. If you, or someone special to you, have this sensitivity, I hope this cookbook will be of help.

It's time to explore and enjoy, ***Caroline's No Nightshade Kitchen: Arthritis Diet.***

THINGS I'VE LEARNED IN THE KITCHEN, AND WANT TO SHARE WITH YOU

Men and women who love to cook also love to share their personal *tricks of the trade.* I do, too. I started cooking when I was eighteen, but it takes a lifetime to craft kitchen skills. Serious cooks never stop learning and sharing what they've learned with friends. Because I now need to cook without nightshades (and without gluten and lactose when cooking for many of my friends), I've learned new tricks that I've shared throughout this cookbook. However, the following tips, suggestions, and basic foods to keep on hand, are a start. Just because some of us need to cook without nightshades, gluten, or lactose, it doesn't mean we have to give up delicious foods and interesting cooking experiences in the kitchen. I hope the following is helpful.

Listen to friends: Your friends are a wealth of information about what and how they cook. Everyone has tips on how to prepare foods faster, better, or what makes their dining choices taste really good. Many of my friends have shared their favorite nightshade, gluten, and lactose free recipes, which are presented throughout this book. Their loving support and contributions were significant to this project. I am grateful for their advice and counsel.

Preserved Lemons: Are you a lemon fan? If you are, once you've tasted preserved lemons in a favorite dish, you'll keep them on hand. My recipe for preserved lemons is located in *Beverages, Sauces, and Other Fun Stuff.* These lemons are easy to prepare and keep in the refrigerator for several months. They are also commercially available in some specialty markets. Add them to ethnic dishes, salads, salad dressings, vegetarian and bean dishes, meats, and fish, etc. They add pizzazz to almost anything.

Stick Blender: This useful device is also called a hand blender, immersion blender, smart stick, or other descriptive name. A stick blender can be used to puree or smooth soups, sauces, etc., and replaces the need to transfer many foods to a food processor or to a traditional blender. Every kitchen needs one of these.

Using a pan for fish on a gas grill: Instead of placing fish directly on the grill rack, I like to grill fish in a shallow container that holds ingredients such as butter, wine, and lemon juice. A flat, metal container lined with foil works well for this purpose. Crimp the corners of the foil and the juices will stay around the fish while it cooks. Because high temperatures from the grill discolor and sometimes warps the pan, I reserve an older pan for this purpose. If you line the pan with foil, followed with a coating of vegetable oil spray so the fish won't stick, the cleanup is easy.

Olive Oil: Olive oil is available in numerous grades and prices. My rule of thumb is to purchase the best products that you can afford. I keep several grades of olive oil on hand, for different uses. Good quality makes a difference in almost everything we eat. However, the highest price is not always the best. Use your own judgment and consider your palate.

Worcestershire Sauce: I've included my version of *Prune Enhanced Worcestershire Sauce* in *Beverages, Sauces, and Other Fun Stuff.* Throughout this book, when I list Worcestershire sauce as an ingredient, I say "Worcestershire without chili extract." The better commercial Worcestershire sauces contain chili extract. If chilies trigger your arthritis, then these products should be avoided. By making the simple recipe found later in this book, you can enjoy a better Worcestershire sauce without nightshades. It's a great condiment for meats and poultry as well.

Keep in the Freezer or Pantry: Toasted oatmeal, almonds, walnuts, and pine nuts are wonderful items to have on hand in the kitchen, as are roasted garlic cloves. Keep the nuts and garlic in individual bags in the freezer, for immediate use the next time your recipe calls for one of these items. Toasted oatmeal, a delicious breakfast option with fruits and yogurt, can be stored in tightly closed containers or zip lock bags in the pantry. Please see *Beverages, Sauces, and Other Fun Stuff,* for simple ways to make these items.

Cornstarch or Arrowroot Substitutes for Flour: I traditionally use flour to thicken many of my recipes, especially sauces and soups. However, when I prepare foods for friends who are gluten intolerant, I substitute cornstarch or arrowroot for the flour. If you're avoiding gluten, substitute one rounded tablespoon of cornstarch or arrowroot (for one rounded tablespoon of flour), mixed in 1/3 cup cold water. Slowly add mixture to the soup or sauce you're preparing and blend well. If additional thickening is needed, repeat step. This formula will vary according to the amount of liquid in your recipe.

Drizzle of Olive Oil: Throughout the following recipes, I often mention *lightly drizzle with olive oil.* I have found that the easiest way to perform this simple task without adding too much oil, is to use a plastic condiment bottle, such as a mustard or catsup dispenser. These can be purchased in most kitchen utensil shops. The spout is small, and usually has a cap. Keep it filled with olive oil, so it's ready when needed.

Black and White Truffle Oils: These fragrant and delicious oils are amazing finishes for eggs, fish, or chicken. Lightly drizzle over prepared foods just before serving. It only takes a few drops. Don't use during the cooking process, as the flavor diminishes with heat. Truffle oils explode with flavor on foods that are ready to serve. Black truffle oils tend to be more pungent than white truffle oils. Keep in the refrigerator after opening.

Tamari vs. Soy Sauce: If you are gluten intolerant, you probably need to avoid regular soy sauce, which contains gluten. Tamari does not contain gluten. Tamari has a richer essence and is often preferred by others who are not affected by gluten but prefer the intense flavor of tamari.

Balsamic Vinegar: Many balsamic vinegars contain gluten. Actually, gluten is found in many of the commercial food items that we eat. If you're gluten intolerant, or you're cooking for someone who is, check ingredient labels carefully of each product you use. Other vinegars that can replace balsamic are: red wine, champagne, white wine, rice, etc.

Caroline's Dry Spicy Rub: As a Southerner, and being partial to barbeque with dry rub, I regretted that I could no longer eat spicy barbeque that contains cayenne and paprika, or any other derivative of the *Solanaceae* (nightshade) family. However, throughout this cookbook, you will find recipes for chicken, fish, and pork that are prepared with *Caroline's Dry Spicy Rub.* My recipe is included in *Beverages, Sauces, and Other Fun Stuff.* Make extra to have on hand for easy suppers cooked on the grill. It's hot and spicy, but contains no nightshades, gluten, or lactose. If you want it hotter, use more rub.

Salt: I use Kosher or sea salts for most of my recipes. A high quality French salt makes an impressive presentation at the table when guests gather, but can also be used during the cooking process. There are endless types, colors, and grades of salt from which to choose, and they are delicious and fun to enjoy. Kosher salt has less salinity than table salt, because of its large, loose structure. Therefore, is less of a concern about over-salting.

Black and White Peppers: I cook abundantly with ground white and black peppers. These peppers are not in the *Solanaceae* (nightshade) plant family, and generally do not cause pain and inflammation for those who suffer with arthritis. Although from the same plant, black pepper is picked while green, then dried in the sun until ripened. White pepper develops completely on the vine. For presentation at the table, place a couple of tablespoons of each ground pepper in a double-sided wasabi and tamari dish. Add a very small serving spoon. White pepper is an intense hot pepper, and is a good substitute for cayenne.

Toasted Sesame Oil: This lovely oil is used in Oriental and Asian cuisines. Both toasted and non-toasted sesame oils are available in most markets, but I prefer the toasted oil. The flavor is greatly enhanced by toasting. Keep this oil refrigerated after opening.

Fresh Herbs: In spring and summer, I grow fresh herbs in my container garden. Of course, they can be purchased throughout the year, but keeping herbs at home during the warmer months is an easy, inexpensive way to have fresh herbs on hand. When it comes to herbs, fresh is the best, but dried herbs can also be flavorful. Purchase dried herbs in small amounts, to shorten their shelf life in your kitchen.

Fresh Garlic and Garlic Flakes: In the following recipes throughout this book, you will find that I sometimes use garlic flakes instead of fresh garlic for specific purposes. However, fresh garlic is the first choice for almost everything I cook. I also roast large amounts of garlic cloves, which I freeze for later use.

Agave substitute for sugar: As a habit of many years, I have avoided sugar. Agave is a good substitute in many of my dessert recipes. Some of the recipes call for sugar, but it's used in minimal amounts, and those recipes are reserved for my guests only.

APPETIZERS FOR FESTIVE STARTS

APPETIZERS FOR FESTIVE STARTS

Appetizers set the tone for a delightful party or evening with friends, and at the same time can be fun to plan and create. In this chapter, there are appetizers for every occasion. Try one of the following recipes at your next brunch, dinner party, holiday event, or cocktail buffet.

Throughout this chapter, preserved lemons are used in many of the recipes. As a reference, a recipe for preserved lemons is found in *Beverages, Sauces, and Other Fun Stuff.*

ITALIAN EGG SALAD

Serves 6-8.

6 hard boiled eggs, coarsely grated
1 stalk celery, minced
½ can flat anchovies, drain slightly and minced
White pepper, to taste
Pinch salt
1 tablespoon Dijon mustard
¼ cup mayonnaise
1 tablespoon onion, grated
1/3 cup Kalamata olives, minced

Mix well and refrigerator for an hour, or longer. Serve on a multi-grain, gluten free crackers, or stuff celery sticks cut in 2 inch pieces.

Nightshade free
Gluten free
Lactose free

GUACAMOLE WITH WASABI

Everyone loves guacamole, but for those who have a nightshade sensitivity to hot peppers and tomatoes, it can be a problem. But, this spicy guac can be made as hot as you like by increasing the wasabi. Enjoy with lime corn chips. Serves 4-6.

2 very ripe avocados, mashed
½ cup black olives, sliced
2 tablespoons grated onion
½ teaspoon Kosher salt
Fresh lime juice, to taste
Wasabi powder or paste, to taste

Place avocados in a bowl, mash until smooth. Add remaining ingredients. Serve immediately, with crisp lime corn chips. Note: To retain green color of avocados, leave seed in mixture until ready to serve.

Nightshade free
Gluten free
Lactose free

EASIEST-BRIE-EVER

Serves 6-8.

Brie
Fresh thyme, minced
Agave

Gently shave the top of Brie, then discard. Sprinkle thyme over the cheese and drizzle agave, to finish. Heat in the microwave until gently warm. Serve with gluten free crackers and slices of apple or pear. (If preferred, use honey, instead of agave.)

Nightshade free
Gluten free

NO... THIS IS THE EASIEST APPETIZER EVER!

Prepare 2-3 servings per guest.

Crisp crackers (gluten free)
Light cream cheese
Preserved lemons

On each cracker, spread approximately 1-2 teaspoons of softened, light cream cheese. Slice a wedge of preserved lemon into thin strips. Place 2 strips in a cross over the cream cheese. Press slightly. Simple, but delicious and elegant! Note: Preserved lemons can be purchased at specialty markets, but a recipe is included in chapter *Beverages, Sauces, and Other Fun Stuff.* They are easy to make, have numerous uses, and keep in the refrigerator for several months.

Nightshade free
Gluten free

ARTICHOKE STEAMED WITH VINAIGRETTE

The magic of springtime artichokes is something to look forward to, and so easy to prepare. They can be served as a first course at dinner, or an appetizer for a cocktail buffet. They're wonderful for patio parties, as well. The vinaigrette is an important finish. One artichoke usually serves 1-2 people.

1-2 large fresh artichokes, trimmed (see below)
Water
Pinch of salt

On a firm surface, lay artichoke on its side. With a serrated knife, trim about 1 inch off top, remove large stem and small leaves, at base. If stickers are present on outer leaves, trim with scissors. Wash well, under running water. Place in a deep pan, with lid, large enough for 1 or 2 artichokes. Add about a 1 ½ inches water and pinch salt, in bottom. Cover and bring to boil. (Use steamer basket if desired, but not necessary.) Reduce heat to full simmer, cover, and cook for about 25-30 minutes, depending on size. When done, place artichoke on cutting board to slightly cool. When ready to serve, push leaves outward with hands, to form a beautiful flower effect. Place on serving plate, drizzle vinaigrette over artichoke, and serve. Include a separate plate to deposit leaves, after guests have eaten and enjoyed tips. IMPORTANT: When guests find the *heart* in bottom of artichoke, take a sharp, small knife and remove any "whiskers" or sharp edges that may be present. Quarter heart for guests to dip in vinaigrette.

SIMPLE VINAIGRETTE
½ cup olive oil
¼ cup red wine vinegar
Kosher salt and pepper, to taste
1 teaspoon dried oregano
½ teaspoon agave, or honey

Whisk ingredients, set aside, until ready to pour over artichoke.

Nightshade free
Gluten free
Lactose free

PRESERVED LEMON CHEESE BALL

For a different variation of the recipe above, **mix 1/3 cup minced preserved lemon into 8 ounces softened light cream cheese.** Form a small, delicious cheese ball. Cross two thin slices of lemon across the top of ball, to garnish. Serve with crisp, gluten free crackers, toast points and/or raw vegetables. Serves 8-10.

Nightshade free
Gluten free

KALE CHIPS WITH LEMON ZEST

Kale appetizers of all kinds are popping up in restaurants, magazines, and in my kitchen. They're over-the-top with flavor, and a healthy boost for any party menu. Preheat oven to 350 degrees. Serves 3-4.

6-8 large kale leaves, stems removed (kale flat, as possible)
1/3 cup olive oil
Kosher salt and black pepper
Zest of 1 lemon

Layer two pieces of parchment paper, on a large cookie sheet. After removing stems from kale, brush each side of leaves with olive oil. Cut kale into 2 inch squares. Place on parchment paper/cookie sheet. Bake for approximately 8 minutes, or until crisp. Remove from oven, zest lemon over pieces. If using multiple trays, halfway through cooking, rotate pans. (Kale reduces in size, when cooked.)

Nightshade free
Gluten free
Lactose free

PROVENCAL SARDINES AND ANCHOVY SPREAD

Several years ago, this recipe was inspired by a dish that was served at a bed and breakfast in Provence, France. The owner included a similar spread on the breakfast buffet with hard cheeses, hard boiled eggs, breads, and jams. It was an interesting change at breakfast, but I especially enjoy this spread as an appetizer with crackers and red wine. Serves 8-10.

2 cans high quality sardines, drained slightly and chopped
2 cans anchovy, drained slightly and minced
1/3 cup olive oil
3 + tablespoons onion, minced
3 + tablespoons garlic, minced
3 + tablespoons fresh parsley, minced

1-2 tablespoons balsamic vinegar
1 -2 tablespoons dried thyme and oregano mixed (or Herbs d' Provence)
Black pepper, to taste
Pinch of salt

Blend well, adjusting seasonings, to taste, and refrigerate for 2-3 hours. Will keep in a tightly closed container for a couple days.

Nightshade free
Lactose free

STEELHEAD OR SALMON TAPAS

Prepare 2-3 servings per guest.

Gluten free cracker
Basil pesto
Steelhead trout or salmon, (seasoned well, cooked, and cut into bite-size pieces)
Avocado slices
Kalamata olives, halved

On each cracker, spread a thin layer of pesto. Top with fish, arrange avocado, and olives on cracker, to finish.

Nightshade free
Gluten free
Lactose free

GREEN PEA AND ROASTED WALNUT HUMMUS

Preheat oven to 350 degrees. Serve with gluten free crackers or raw vegetables. Serves 6-8.

1/3 cup toasted walnuts
1/3 cup roasted garlic cloves

2 cups frozen green peas, cooked and drained
Kosher salt and black pepper, to taste
1-2 tablespoon onion, minced
1 ½ teaspoons dry mustard
4 tablespoons preserved lemon, chopped
(or juice of 1 lemon, and zest of 1 lemon)
6 tablespoons olive oil

In preheated oven, roast/toast walnuts and garlic cloves (in the same small pan lined with foil), for 11-12 minutes. If the walnuts cook faster than the garlic, remove walnuts and continue to roast garlic. Place all ingredients in a food processor, and pulse to puree, but leave some texture. Chill 1-2 hours. Serve at room temperature.

Nightshade free
Gluten free
Lactose free

ARTICHOKE FETA RELISH

Serves 4.

¾ cup oil packed artichoke hearts, coarsely chopped
½ cup feta
3-4 tablespoons capers
1 tablespoon onion, grated
½ cup black olives, sliced
1-2 tablespoons olive oil
Crushed black peppercorns, to taste

Mix all ingredients well. Refrigerate for 1 hour. Serve chilled or at room temperature, with gluten free crackers.

Nightshade free
Gluten free

SARDINE AND APPLE SPREAD

Present with gluten free crackers and raw vegetables, as an appetizer. Serves 8.

3 tablespoons onion, minced
1-2 garlic cloves, minced
½ cup mayonnaise
1 apple, unpeeled, cored, and diced
3 tablespoons Dijon mustard
2 hard boiled eggs, diced
2 tablespoons fresh lemon juice
2 cans high quality sardines, drained

Mix onion, garlic, mayonnaise, apple, mustard, eggs, and lemon. Break sardines in to bite size pieces, add to other ingredients, and toss lightly, being careful not to mash.

Nightshade free
Gluten free
Lactose free

TAPENADE

Serves 6.

½ lb. mix of favorite olives, drained and pitted (none with pimento stuffing)
½ cup capers, drained
½ can anchovies
4-5 tablespoons olive oil
1-2 tablespoon fresh lemon juice
Lots of coarse black pepper, or to taste

Pulse in food processor until mixed well, but leave chunky. Serve with crackers, or use in pasta dishes.

Nightshade free
Gluten free
Lactose free

CAROLINE'S DEVILED EGGS...TWO WAYS

Perfect not only during the Easter season, but for picnics, cocktail buffets, or other occasion when finger foods are front stage. Serves 8-10.

1 dozen eggs, hard boiled, peeled, and halved
1 can anchovies, slightly drained and minced
½ cup mayonnaise, or more
1 tablespoon yellow mustard
2 tablespoons sweet relish (without red peppers)
Salt and white pepper, to taste

Gently remove the yokes from the eggs, placing outer whites on a large platter. Place the yokes in a bowl. Mash with other ingredients, until fluffy, using a fork. Add additional mayonnaise, if needed. Spoon the mixture into the center of the whites. The finished eggs can be garnished with a slice of olive, sweet pickle, or fresh parsley.

ANOTHER VERSION:
1 dozen eggs, hard boiled, peeled, and halved
1 can anchovies, slightly drained and minced
½ cup mayonnaise, or more
1 tablespoon yellow mustard
½ cup cilantro, coarsely chopped
3 tablespoons onion, finely minced
Salt and white pepper, to taste

Mix the ingredients for the version above, fill egg whites. Garnishes are not recommended for this recipe, as the cilantro adds color and texture.

Nightshade free
Gluten free
Lactose free

LEMON HUMMUS

Serves 8-10.

2 cans garbanzo beans, rinsed and drained
6-8 cloves garlic, coarsely chopped
1/3 cup tahini
3 tablespoons preserved lemon, coarsely chopped (or to taste)
¾ cup olive oil
½ teaspoon cumin
Kosher salt, to taste
White pepper, to taste

Blend all ingredients until smooth in a food processor. Add additional olive oil, for desired consistency. Adjust seasonings.

Nightshade free
Gluten free
Lactose free

SMOKED SALMON ON THE GRILL

Serves 10 as appetizer, or 6 as main course.

3 to 5 lb. filet of salmon, rinsed and dried
1 ½ cup water
½ cup brown sugar
6 tablespoons Kosher or sea salt
1 tablespoon ground ginger
1 teaspoon allspice, optional
3-4 bay leaves
Black peppercorns
Honey

In a medium sauce pan, combine water, brown sugar, salt, ginger, allspice (optional), and bay leaves. Bring to a gentle boil, cool slightly. Pour over the fish in a large container, preferably with cover, and store in refrigerator for 4-8 hours. The longer the fish marinates, the higher the salt flavor and content. When ready to smoke, remove the fish from the marinate and place in a heavy *foil boat* that will stabilize the fish while smoking. Press black peppercorns into flesh of fish. Discard marinade. Preheat gas grill to 300 degrees, with fire under one side only. When grill is hot, place a cup of water soaked wood chips, on hot side of grill. Have additional wet chips available, for later use. Place the salmon, in foil boat, on cool side of grill. Close grill lid and smoke for approximately 2-3 hours, depending on size of fish. Control temperature to maintain 300 degrees by venting lid, if necessary. Fish will become firm with a rich, brown color. When done, let salmon cool slightly, then drizzle a couple tablespoons of honey over fish. Serve immediately, or store in refrigerator when cool.

Nightshade free
Gluten free
Lactose free

MEDITERRANEAN FETA

This recipe is simple and you can add or omit items, as you choose. The more ingredients you use, the more complex the flavors. Serve with gluten free crackers. Serves 4-6.

¼-½ pound feta cheese
¼-½ pound pitted Kalamata olives, sliced
1-2 tablespoon capers
½ + cup artichoke hearts, quartered
1 teaspoon dried thyme
½ teaspoon dried oregano
½ teaspoon dried rosemary
2 tablespoons mint, fresh and minced
2 tablespoons preserved lemons, minced

½ teaspoon garlic flakes
Pinch salt
½ teaspoon black pepper
1 tablespoon fresh parsley, minced
Olive oil, as needed

Arrange and layer items in a tightly covered container, fill with olive oil. Invert several times to distribute seasonings. Refrigerate one hour, but serve at room temperature.

Nightshade free
Gluten free

LAYERED RICE PESTO TORTE

Preheat oven to 400 degrees. Serves 12.

Vegetable oil spray
3 cups Calzone rice, cooked
2 cups Parmesan cheese
¼ cup Parmesan cheese (additional for topping)
Salt, white and black peppers, to taste
1 ½ to 2 cups basil pesto, divided
½ cup pine nuts, divided
1 cup black olives, thinly sliced and divided
4-6 oz. goat cheese, crumbled and divided

Coat 7-inch springform pan with vegetable oil spray. In a large bowl, combine the cooked rice, 2 cups Parmesan cheese, salt and peppers, to taste. Blend well. Place half the rice mixture in bottom of springform pan, patting down. Place half the pesto evenly over the rice, followed by half the goat cheese, half the pine nuts, and half the black olives. Repeat layer, then sprinkle an additional ¼ cup Parmesan on top. Bake for 20-25 minutes, or until heated thoroughly. Remove sides of springform after placing pan on serving platter. (The pesto provides moisture to maintain shape of torte.) Serve at room temperature.

Nightshade free

Gluten free

STUFFING-STUFFED MUSHROOMS

When you are nearly finished with the leftover stuffing at Thanksgiving, freeze 2 cups for stuffing mushrooms during the Christmas holidays. Here's how. Preheat oven to 350 degrees. Serves 8-10.

18-24 white mushrooms
2 cups leftover stuffing
3 tablespoons Parmesan cheese, grated
Olive oil

As you remove the stems of the mushrooms, scoop additional flesh from the center below the stem. Place mushrooms on a large cookie sheet. Fill each with stuffing, sprinkle with cheese, slightly drizzle with olive oil. Bake until mushrooms are done. Serve hot.

Nightshade free

BLUE CHEESE CROSTINI

Simple and a prize! Prepare 2-3 servings per guest.
Layer each appetizer in the following order:

1. **Slice and toast baguette (or use gluten free cracker)**
2. **Spread of softened blue cheese**
3. **Drop of honey**
4. **Two drops truffle oil**

Nightshade free

PESTO AND SUMMER SAUSAGE ON CRACKER

Prepare 2 servings per guest. Layer each appetizer in the following in order:

1. **Crisp cracker (gluten free)**
2. **Two narrow strips summer sausage, crossed**
3. **½ teaspoon pesto**
4. **3-4 pine nuts**

Nightshade free
Gluten free
Lactose free

SALMON CUCUMBER APPETIZER

Serves 8-10.

1. **Mix 8 ounces softened light cream cheese with wasabi powder or paste, to taste.**
2. **Spread cheese mixture on gluten free cracker.**
3. **Place a thin slice of English cucumber on cheese.**
4. **Top with thin slices of avocado and/or smoked salmon.**

Nightshade free
Gluten free

ARTICHOKE, TUNA, AND SPINACH DIP

Preheat oven to 375 degrees. Serves 12.

2 6.5 oz. cans tuna, drained
14 oz. oil packed artichokes, drained and chopped
½ cup light sour cream
¾ - 1 cup mayonnaise
2 tablespoons Dijon mustard
Dash tamari
1 cup frozen spinach, thaw and squeezed dry

½ cup Parmesan cheese, grated
½ + teaspoon white pepper, to taste

Mix all ingredients well. Add additional mayonnaise, if needed. Place in a small casserole. Heat thoroughly for approximately 20 minutes, or until hot.

Nightshade free
Gluten free

CUCUMBER SANDWICHES

This spread has been a main-stay at my parties since the 1970s.
Serves 8-10.

8 oz. light cream cheese, softened
½ sweet onion, minced
1 medium cucumber, peeled, seeded, and chopped
½ to 3/4 cup mayonnaise
Salt and white pepper, to taste
White bread or crisp crackers (gluten free)

Blend the ingredients well. Add additional mayonnaise, as needed. For finger sandwiches, spread on white bread triangles or quarters, with crust removed. Or, serve as a dip with crisp crackers and mixed raw vegetables.

Nightshade free
Gluten free

SWEET POTATO AND HORSERADISH PATE

Sweet potatoes are perfect in many recipes when you're looking for something that is unusual and is nightshade, gluten, and lactose free. This pate is a lovely first course at dinner or a luncheon, but can also be served with gluten free crackers at a cocktail buffet. See suggested presentation as a first course below. Serves 10-15.

1-2 large sweet potatoes, peeled and sliced

Kosher salt, black and white peppers, to taste
½ cup mayonnaise
3 hard boiled eggs, diced
1/3 cup onion, minced
2 tablespoons fresh lemon juice
1 cup celery, small diced
Horseradish, to taste
Red lettuce leaves
Black olives, sliced
Celery sticks, cut in 2 -3 inch pieces

Boil sweet potatoes with dash of salt and black pepper, until tender, about 20 minutes. Drain and set aside. While potatoes are warm, add mayonnaise, eggs, onion, lemon juice, and diced celery, mixing well. Place in refrigerator. Chill thoroughly, then add horseradish, white and black peppers, to desired taste. To serve as a first course, place 1 lettuce leaf on each salad plate, adding about ½ cup potato pate in a rounded ball. (Pate should be slightly stiff, to maintain shape in this presentation.) Add a celery stick in top of pate, with 2-3 sliced black olives, as garnish. Serve immediately.

Nightshade free
Gluten free
Lactose free

SURPRISING PIZZAS

Don't miss **SURPRISING PIZZAS**, which follows in this cookbook. Any of these pizzas, cut into 2 inch squares, make delicious additions to cocktail buffets, or appetizers before a dinner party.

SUCCULENT SOUPS AND STEWS

SUCCULENT SOUPS AND STEWS

Summer or winter, soups and stews are a tradition at my table. Just the thought of soup makes me smile.

On a blazing hot summer's day, I want a chilled soup that is icy cold, but is rich in flavor, such as *Watermelon Gazpacho*. If snow is piling up outside my window, I want a hearty ragout, like *Italian Country Stew,* that will warm and comfort. This chapter contains Asian, Italian, French, Greek, African, Indian, Russian, Thai, Persian, and *good ole American recipes.* Hot and cold options are sprinkled throughout this chapter.

Soups and Stews can be the main event at a dinner party, but also, are excellent choices at other times. Why not serve *Egg Drop Soup* at your next brunch, paired with a favorite vegetable strata. When you think about soup or stew, think about the endless, delicious recipes that can be created from almost anything. Making soup is an adventure filled with rich flavors.

CANTALOUPE, ONION, AND CUCUMBER GAZPACHO WITH ORANGE

For something different, spicy, and refreshing on a hot summer's day, try this nightshade and gluten free cold soup. If you want to tame the spice, reduce white pepper. Serves 4-5.

1 cantaloupe, seeded and diced
1 cucumber, peeled and diced
½ onion, minced
2-3 green scallions, sliced
Zest of l lemon

Juice of 1 lemon
3 tablespoons white wine vinegar
1 teaspoon white pepper, or to taste
¼ teaspoon black pepper
Salt, to taste
1 teaspoon dried basil
¼ cup fresh mint, minced
2 cups yogurt
1 cup ice cold water
2 cups orange juice

Place first 12 ingredients in a large mixing bowl. Blend well, slowly add yogurt, until smooth. Add cold water and orange juice. Mix well, and chill for several hours.

Nightshade free
Gluten free

SHRIMP AND SWEET POTATO BISQUE

While in Pensacola, Florida on vacation, I enjoyed a sweet potato bisque at a local restaurant, which inspired *Shrimp and Sweet Potato Bisque.* By adding shrimp and several other ingredients, this soup became an elegant, spicy main course. Serves 6.

2 large sweet potatoes, peeled and sliced
Salt and black pepper, to taste
3+ tablespoons olive oil
1 large leek, washed carefully, dried, and coarsely chopped
3 garlic cloves, minced
10 large raw shrimp (or more)
1-2 teaspoon white pepper, or to taste
¼ cup brandy
½ cup Madeira sherry

½ stick butter
¼ cup all purpose flour
2 cups half and half (or 2% milk)
4-6 cups seafood broth
Chives or parsley, and sour cream, to garnish

In a medium pot, cook the sweet potatoes covered in water, with salt and pepper, for approximately 30 minutes. Drain, and set aside. In a large pot or Dutch oven, add 3 tablespoons of olive oil, sauté the leek and garlic until soft, for approximately 8-10 minutes. Add shrimp and 1 teaspoon of white pepper and ½ teaspoon salt. Cook for 2 minutes, turning shrimp once. Add brandy and Madeira sherry, cooking 3 minutes more, or until shrimp turn pink. Transfer the shrimp mixture and drained sweet potatoes to a food processor. Process in batches, but leave some texture. It may be necessary to add seafood broth, to thin as you process. Place sweet potato/shrimp mixture in a bowl, set aside. In the same large pot, melt ½ stick butter. Heat until bubbly, add flour. Whisk mixture, while adding half and half. Continue to whisk, until mixture begins to slightly thicken. Slowly blend. Whisk shrimp, sweet potato, and leek puree into half and half mixture. Continue mixing, while slowly adding seafood stock. Use additional stock, as desired for consistency. Test seasonings. Heat thoroughly, but do not boil. Garnish with sour cream, chopped chives, or sprig of parsley.

Nightshade free

CUCUMBER AND YOGURT SOUP

Good friend and cook, Dasha, recommends this luscious Persian soup for hot summer days. The flavors are enchanting, cooling, and the raisins add a touch of sweetness. Perfect for a luncheon or supper on the porch.

Serves 4-6.

½ cup golden raisins (or more)
2-3 cups low fat yogurt

½ cup light cream (or 2 % lactose free milk)
6 ice cubes
1 cucumber, peeled, seeded, and diced
¼ cup green onions
2 teaspoons salt
½ teaspoon black pepper, or to taste
1 cup cold water
2 tablespoons fresh parsley, minced (garnish)
2 tablespoon fresh dill, minced (garnish)
1-2 eggs, hard boiled (see note below)

Soak raisins in cold water for 5 minutes, to soften, drain well. Place yogurt in a large bowl (or plastic container, with lid). Add raisins, cream/milk, ice cubes, cucumber, green onions, salt, and pepper. Add 1 cup cold water, mixing well. Refrigerate, covered for 2-3 hours, or up to 1 day. Garnish with parsley and dill. NOTE: The eggs can be diced, added to the soup before chilling. Or, if preferred, slice eggs, place pieces in center of each bowl of soup, with other garnishes.

Nightshade free
Gluten free

GREEK (AVGOLEMONO) SOUP

This luscious soup is the perfect remedy when you or a friend have a cold. Serves 6-8.

8 cups chicken stock
½ cup uncooked rice
5 egg yolks
2-3 tablespoons preserved lemon, minced
1 ½ cups frozen green peas
1 ½ cups frozen corn
1 7-10 oz. can of white chicken, with liquid (optional)

White pepper and salt, to taste
Fresh spinach leaves (optional)

Bring chicken stock to a boil. Pour in rice, and simmer for 25 minutes. In a bowl, beat egg yolks until smooth and creamy. Pour about ½ cup hot broth into the egg mixture, stirring constantly. Pour egg/mix back into the broth, blending well. Add preserved lemons. Add the frozen corn, peas, and chicken, if desired. Simmer until vegetables are tender. Season with white pepper and salt, to taste. To thin soup, add additional chicken stock or hot water. As an option, add spinach leaves to hot soup, before serving.

Nightshade free
Gluten free
Lactose free

CRAB AND ASPARAGUS SOUP

My friend, Dasha, shared this outstanding recipe. Fresh asparagus brings French influence to the soup, which marries well with the Vietnamese flavors. I added additional asparagus and mushrooms, for texture.

Serves 3-4.

1 ½ cup dried mushroom mix, dehydrated
(or mix of fresh mushrooms)
8 oz. crab meat, flaked
1 qt. chicken stock
1 tablespoon cornstarch (in 1/3 cup cold water)
1 egg, beaten
1 ½ cups fresh asparagus, cut on diagonal
Kosher or sea salt, and black pepper, to taste
8 quail eggs, hard boiled (optional)
Cilantro and black pepper

Soak mushrooms in water for about 30 minutes to rehydrate, squeeze dry, then coarsely chop. Add crabmeat and mushrooms to chicken stock, and bring to boil. Simmer for about 20-30 minutes, or until mushrooms soften. Gradually add cornstarch mixture to soup, followed by the beaten egg. Mix well. Add asparagus, and season to taste. Cook gently for 3 minutes. Serve hot, topping each portion with 2 quail eggs (optional). Finish with chopped cilantro and black pepper.

Nightshade free
Gluten free
Lactose free

AFRICAN PEANUT SOUP

This spicy, fragrant soup is a *no-nightshade* version of one of my all-time favorite soups, which previously contained red and green bell peppers, tomatoes, and cayenne. The *spicy level* in this recipe is determined by the amount of white and black peppers used. White pepper can be as hot as cayenne. Please adjust to your palate. Serves 4.

2 tablespoons olive oil
1 cup sweet onion, chopped
2 carrots, thinly sliced
1 sweet potato, diced
3 garlic cloves, minced
1 teaspoon salt
1 teaspoon black pepper
1 teaspoon white pepper (more, for additional heat)
2 tablespoons fresh ginger, minced (Thai ginger, preferred)
2 cups water
4 cups chicken stock
½ cup chunky peanut butter
¾ cup half and half

In a soup pot, sauté the onion in olive oil, until translucent. Add carrots, sweet potato, garlic, salt, black and white peppers, ginger, water, and chicken stock. Bring to boil, simmer for about 30 minutes uncovered. The liquid will reduce as the soup simmers, melding the flavors. When the vegetables are very tender, place in a food processor in batches, with the peanut butter. Blend until smooth, return to the soup pot. (If using a stick blender, process in soup pot.) Bring to a gentle boil, reduce heat, add half and half. Mix well, adjust seasoning before serving. Note: Thai ginger has a very spicy flavor, which adds greatly to this soup.

Nightshade free

Gluten free

PUREE OF ROASTED CABBAGE AND ONION SOUP WITH APPLE

A recipe for *Roasted Cabbage* is found in *Lovely Vegetables and Vegetarian Entrees.* When you prepare that recipe, roast extra vegetables that can be saved for the following soup. The caramelized vegetables are key to this soup. Serves 6.

4 cups roasted cabbage and onions (seasoned as described in original recipe)

1 apple, cored, diced, with skin

2 cups fresh spinach

1 qt. chicken stock

Water

Butter

Kosher salt and black pepper, to taste

Light sour cream and parsley, to garnish

Place roasted cabbage/onion mix, apple, spinach, and chicken stock, in a large pot, with lid. Add water, to cover contents 1 inch above ingredients. Bring to boil, simmer slightly covered, for approximately 30-45 minutes, or until apple is tender. Add water, if needed. Cool slightly. Puree soup in a food processor, or use a stick blender in soup pot. Return soup to boil, add butter, salt and pepper, as desired. Garnish with a dollop of sour cream and pinch of parsley.

Nightshade free

Gluten free

Lactose free (omit butter and sour cream)

PUREE OF SOUTHWEST VEGETABLE SOUP WITH LIME AND AVOCADO

Here's another special soup that is pureed to a smooth consistency. Once again, roasting the vegetables is key, but the southwest flavors greatly enhance this soup. Preheat oven to 375 degrees. Serves 4-6.

ROASTING VEGETABLES:
½ head of green cabbage
12-15 whole garlic cloves
3 small sweet potatoes, peeled and sliced
2 cups small carrots
1 cup onion, sliced
2 cups Brussels sprouts, trimmed and halved
1 cup celery, sliced
Olive oil
Kosher salt, pepper, and dried oregano

On a foil lined large cookie sheet, arrange vegetables, drizzle with olive oil. Follow with salt, pepper, and dried oregano. In preheated oven, roast for approximately 1 hour, or until slightly browned and very tender. Place vegetables in a large pot, with the following ingredients:

1 qt. chicken stock
Water, as needed
1-2 teaspoons cumin, to taste
Kosher salt and pepper, to taste

1-3 limes (save 1 lime for garnish)
Avocados, sliced for garnish

Bring to boil, simmer for about 45 minutes. Cool slightly. Puree mixture with a stick blender in pot, or use a food processor. When very smooth, reheat soup. Season with cumin, salt and pepper, as needed, and juice of 1 or more limes. Serve in soup bowls, with slices of avocado and lime wedges.

Nightshade free
Gluten free
Lactose free

FRENCH ONION SOUP

Always a favorite at our house, this soup is better the next day. In traditional French Onion soup recipes, the onions are typically caramelized slowly, for 30-40 minutes, so not to brown. My friend Bo, made this soup, but browned the onions. When I saw the rich golden color of his soup, and tasted the enhanced flavors, I adopted his method. Serves 8.

Stick of butter
8-9 large sweet onions, sliced and halved
1 quart of beef stock
1 quart of chicken stock
Madeira sherry, to taste
Salt, black and white peppers, to taste
1 tablespoon thyme, dried
1-2 tablespoon oregano, dried
1-2 tablespoons cornstarch and 1/3 cup cold water, optional
1 ½ cups Swiss cheese, grated
1 cup Parmesan cheese, grated
Italian bread, cut in ¾ inch slices

Place butter and onions, in large stock pot. Bring to high heat, reduce to medium. Sauté onions for approximately 20-30 minutes, stirring often.

When the onions are golden brown in color, add beef and chicken stocks, 1 cup Madeira sherry, salt, both peppers, thyme, and oregano. Bring to a boil, simmer for 30-40 minutes. Adjust seasonings, including herbs and Madeira, as desired. (Note: To thicken soup slightly, mix 1-2 tablespoons cornstarch with 1/3 cup cold water. Add slowly to pot, while simmering.) Toast Italian bread slices, with ample amounts of both cheeses. Pour soup into large bowls. Partially submerge cheese toast into soup. Serve hot.

Nightshade free

Gluten free (Use gluten free bread)

CREAMED ENGLISH PEAS AND ONION SOUP

Smooth and creamy, but without cream. Serve as a first course at dinner, or with a salad at a luncheon. Serves 4.

4 onions, thinly sliced
Vegetable oil spray
3-4 tablespoons butter
2 cups 1% or 2% milk (or more as needed)
2 heaping tablespoons cornstarch
2 cups frozen (or fresh) green peas
1 tablespoon dried tarragon
Kosher salt and white pepper, to taste

Place thinly sliced onions in bottom of a medium pan, coated with vegetable oil spray and 2 tablespoons butter (or more, if needed while cooking). Saute for approximately 20-25 minutes, until very soft, but not browned. Add cornstarch to ½ cup cold milk, mixing well. Add to onions. As onions begin to thicken, slowly add milk, for desired consistency. Add more milk, if needed. When bubbly, add peas and cook until tender, over low heat. Add tarragon, salt and pepper, to taste.

Nightshade free

Gluten free

BEER CHEESE SOUP

My daughter, Claire, enjoys this luscious soup, but her version is not only nightshade free, but the calorie count is reduced. This soup stands alone, or can be served with crusty French bread. Another great soup for football Sundays. Serves 6.

7 ribs celery, chopped
7 medium carrots, chopped
1 small white onion, chopped
4 oz. light butter
2 cans fat free chicken stock
2 cans cream of celery soup, with 2 cans of low-fat milk
8 oz. light sour cream
8 oz. Kraft Velveeta Cheese (reduced-fat), cubed
Bottle beer
Popcorn, garnish

Place celery, carrots, onion, and butter, in a soup pot. Saute until vegetables are tender, approximately 10 minutes. Add 2 cans of chicken stock, bring to boil. Add 2 cans of cream of celery soup, with 2 cans milk. Stir until blended, simmer about 15 minutes. Add sour cream, mixing until blended. Add a few cubes of cheese at a time, to hot mixture, stirring constantly. When melted, add beer. Simmer 10-15 minutes. Garnish with popcorn, serve immediately.

Nightshade free
Gluten free

BLACK BEAN SOUP WITH TOPPINGS

Black bean soup is a favorite in many kitchens, and certainly is in mine. This is one of the soups that I changed early on, when I discovered I needed to eliminate nightshades from my diet. My original recipe contained red pepper flakes, bell pepper, and cayenne. It no longer does, and neither do the toppings that I include on the serving buffet. Serves 4-6.

16 oz. package black beans,
washed, picked over, and soaked overnight
1 large onion, diced
5-6 large garlic cloves, minced
4 tablespoons olive oil
1 qt. chicken or beef broth, or combination
(have extra quart on hand, as soup simmers)
Kosher salt and black pepper, to taste
White pepper, to taste
2 tablespoons oregano, dried
1 tablespoon parsley, dried
1-2 teaspoons dried rosemary, crushed
Madeira sherry
Water, as needed

Drain soaked black beans, rinse again, and drain. Place in a large soup pot. Add onion and garlic, with olive oil, and saute to caramelize. Add remaining ingredients, except Madeira and water. Bring to a boil, reduce heat, cover, and simmer about 1 ½ hours, or until beans are very tender. While cooking, add additional chicken/beef stock, as needed (and water if necessary), but control liquids for desired consistency. (The soup should be fluid, but slightly thick.) When soup is done, add 1 cup Madeira and bring to boil. Adjust seasonings, herbs, and Madeira, adding as needed. This final adjustment is an important step. Cool slightly. Puree soup in a food processor, in batches if necessary, but leave some texture. If using a stick blender, puree in soup pot. Reheat before serving. Note: Prepare selections of the following toppings in small bowls. Place toppings around the crock of black bean soup on the serving buffet for guests to serve themselves.

TOPPINGS:
Light sour cream or Greek yogurt
Grated cheese(s)
Sliced green onions

Sliced avocados
Browned ground sirloin, well seasoned
Cilantro, roughly chopped
Black olives, sliced
Brown or white rice, cooked and seasoned

Nightshade free
Gluten free
Lactose free (omit dairy toppings)

EGG DROP SOUP

Serves 6 appetizer soups.

6 cups chicken stock
1 cup frozen green peas
Salt and white pepper, to taste
1-2 tablespoons preserved lemon, minced
(or 3 tablespoons fresh lemon juice)
4-5 eggs, well beaten

Bring chicken stock to a rapid boil. As stock continues to boil, add green peas, salt, pepper, and preserved lemons. Simmer until peas are done. Slowly pour beaten eggs into broth, stirring in a whirling motion. When eggs have set, adjust seasonings, and serve.

Nightshade free
Gluten free
Lactose free

CHICKEN STEW WITH SPRING VEGETABLES FOR PASSOVER

This lovely stew was adapted from a traditional Passover recipe, which incorporates seasonal vegetables. The soup, without the chicken, can be served as a first course during the Seder, or a main course stew during Passover Week. Once again, this modified recipe is nightshade, gluten and lactose free. Serves 6.

1 ½ lbs. chicken breasts, with bone
1 ½ lbs. chicken thighs or drumsticks
1 large onion, sliced
1 bay leaf
4 sprigs fresh thyme (or ½ teaspoon dried)
Approximately 2 quarts water
4-5 medium carrots, in 2 inch slices
1 lb. asparagus, sliced in 2 inch slices
Kosher salt and pepper, to taste
½ cup green scallions, sliced

Place chicken in a large Dutch oven or pot, with lid. Add onion, bay leaf, and thyme. Cover with ample water. Bring to a boil. Skim foam, as necessary. Cover and simmer 1 hour. Add carrots, simmer covered, for 45 minutes. Remove bay leaf and thyme sprigs. Remove skin from chicken and bone meat. Return to pot. Reheat soup. Add asparagus and cook 10 minutes. Season with salt and pepper, to taste. Stir in green scallions and serve in large bowls.

Nightshade free
Gluten free
Lactose free

ITALIAN COUNTRY STEW

This hearty, fragrant stew, serves 10.

3 tablespoons olive oil
1 large onion, chopped
2 skinless/boneless chicken breasts (sliced in ½ inch pieces)
2 quarts chicken stock (plus water, as needed)
2 stalks celery, sliced
2 carrots, sliced
7-8 mushrooms, sliced
1 zucchini, sliced
4 garlic cloves, minced
2 cans white kidney beans, rinsed and drained
1 can black beans, rinsed and drained
2 teaspoon basil, dried
2 teaspoon oregano, dried
Kosher salt, white and black peppers, to taste
2 tablespoons preserved lemon, minced
(or 3 tablespoons fresh lemon juice)
½ -3/4 cup dry vermouth
1 cup Kalamata olives
Can black olives, drained
Garnishes: yogurt, cilantro, and feta

Sauté onions in olive oil. Add all ingredients, except vermouth, olives, and garnishes. Bring to a boil, reduce heat and simmer 30 minutes, slightly covered. Before serving, add vermouth and olives. Adjust seasonings. Pass garnishes at table.

Nightshade free
Gluten free
Lactose free (omit cheese)

WATERMELON GAZPACHO

This soup was inspired by a recipe in *Gourmet Magazine Cookbook.* Serve this summer treat as a first course at dinner, or main course at a luncheon. This flavorful cold soup is an alternative to traditional gazpachos, which often contain tomatoes and peppers. Serves 4-6.

4 pound seedless watermelon (flesh scooped out to make 7 cups)
1 ½ cups ice cubes
1 cup whole roasted almonds
3-4 garlic cloves, coarsely chopped
6-8 sliced Italian white bread slices,
with crust and torn into pieces
2-3 tablespoons red wine vinegar
2 teaspoons Kosher or sea salt
½ - 1 teaspoon coarse black pepper, or to taste
White pepper, to taste, but optional
¼ cup olive oil

In a blender, puree watermelon flesh in batches. You may need a large bowl to reserve puree. Puree will have a slight texture. Blend watermelon puree with ice, almonds, and garlic, in batches as necessary, until smooth. (A stick blender is NOT recommended for this recipe.) Add bread, vinegar, salt and pepper, to taste, blend again. While motor is running, add oil in a slow pour thru top of blender lid. Mix all ingredients well, until smooth. Serve immediately, or chill for a couple hours. This chilled soup is best served the same day.

Nightshade free
Lactose free

MULLIGATAWNY SOUP

In the mid-seventies, I was first introduced to the incredible flavors of this traditional Indian soup, in Memphis, Tennessee. The soup enchanted me, but over time, the nightshades that originally filled my soup bowl, caused severe pain in my hands. Here's Mulligatawny soup *without nightshades*, but the flavors remain rich and delicious. Note: This soup is best when refrigerated a few hours, then reheated. Serves 6-8.

6 tablespoons butter (two uses)
2 medium carrots, sliced
2 medium onions, chopped
4 garlic cloves, chopped
2 medium sweet potatoes, diced
7 cups chicken stock
2 cups spinach, packed tightly
1 cup roasted almonds
1 cup water
¼ teaspoon saffron and 2 tablespoons water
4 teaspoons mild yellow curry
(containing no cayenne or paprika)
1 can light unsweetened coconut milk
½ cup cilantro, chopped
Kosher salt, to taste
1 teaspoon black pepper, to taste
2 teaspoon white pepper, or more
Greek yogurt and extra cilantro (garnishes)

In a large soup pot, melt butter, add carrots, onions, garlic, and sweet potatoes. Cook about 10 minutes, stirring to heat vegetables. Add chicken stock, bring to boil, simmer for approximately 25-30 minutes, or until vegetables are soft. Add spinach leaves, and cook 2-3 minutes longer. Puree the mixture until smooth. (I use a *stick blender*, instead of a food processor or regular blender, for this procedure.) Return to heat. In *regular blender*, combine almonds and water, to make almond milk. (Do not use stick blender for this step.) Process until smooth, but a little crunchy. Set aside. Place saffron and water in small container, for 15 minutes. In small sauce pan, add 2 tablespoons butter and mild yellow curry. Cook over medium heat, until fragrance is released, about 2 minutes. Add curry, almond milk, and saffron water to soup, mixing well. Stir in light unsweetened coconut milk and chopped cilantro. Season with salt, white and black peppers, to taste. White pepper adds the spicy flavors needed for this soup. Serve with a garnish of cilantro. Pass Greek yogurt, at the table.

Nightshade free
Gluten free
Lactose free (omit Greek yogurt)

HEARTY LENTIL SOUP

Serves 6

2-3 tablespoons olive oil
1 cup onion, chopped
4-5 garlic cloves, minced
1 ½ cups mushroom, sliced
1 cup carrot, sliced
1 ½ cups celery, sliced
½ cup ham, minced
1 teaspoon dried rosemary
1 teaspoon dried sage
1 teaspoon thyme
Salt and pepper, to taste
1 tablespoon preserved lemon, minced
16 oz. dried lentils, washed and picked over
1 quart chicken stock
2 - 4 cups water, as needed

In a large pot, add olive oil and vegetables, increase heat. When onion and garlic caramelize, and the other vegetables become hot, add ham, herbs, salt, pepper, preserved lemon, and lentils. Mix well, add chicken stock, and 2-3 cups of water. Add additional water, as needed during cooking process. Bring to a boil, slightly cover, reduce heat to simmer. Cook approximately 45 minutes, or until lentils are tender. Adjust seasonings.

Nightshade free
Gluten free
Lactose free

BORSCHT

Serve borscht steaming hot, as a radiant addition to your Christmas feast. The rich color of this soup steals the show! However, borscht is just as special on a hot summer's day, thoroughly chilled. As a garnish for summer borscht, pass horseradish at the table. Serves 8-10.

4 large beets, peeled and diced
2 medium sweet potatoes, peeled and diced
2 ribs celery, sliced
1 large onion, chopped
4 garlic cloves, minced
Water
Kosher salt and black pepper, to taste
4 cups chicken stock
3 tablespoons white wine vinegar
2 teaspoons dill weed
Light sour cream

Place beets, sweet potatoes, celery, onion, and garlic in a large pot. Cover with water. Lightly season with salt and pepper. Bring to a boil, reduce to a full simmer for 45 minutes, or until tender. Keep water level slightly covering vegetables at all times. Cool for a few minutes. Puree vegetables (with some of the water), using a stick blender or food processor, until smooth. Add chicken stock (4 cups, or for desired consistency), white wine vinegar, and dill weed. Bring to a simmer to heat thoroughly. Season with additional salt and black pepper, as needed. Place hot soup in serving bowls with a dollop of sour cream in center, and sprinkle of dill weed. (To serve cold, refrigerator for several hours or overnight.)

Nightshade free
Gluten free
Lactose free (omit sour cream)

NEW ENGLAND CLAM CHOWDER

Serves 6 as first course.

1 - 51 ounce can chopped sea clams, drain with juice reserved (approximately 3 cups juice)
1 bottle commercial clam juice, if needed
1 large shallot, minced
3 ribs celery, minced
4-5 tablespoons butter
3 tablespoons flour
3 cups parsnips and carrot mix, peeled and diced
1 quart (total) 2 % milk/half and half mix
Salt and white pepper, to taste
3 tablespoons fresh parsley, minced
2 tablespoons butter, to finish (optional)

Drain clams and reserve juice. Set aside. Sauté shallot and celery in butter, until tender. Slowly add flour, stirring for 3 minutes. Add reserved clam juice, whisk to blend. Include bottle clam juice, if needed. Add parsnips and carrots to pot, mixing well. Bring to a gentle boil, then simmer until vegetables are tender, approximately 10 -12 minutes. Add minimal water if necessary, while cooking vegetables. Add clams, with milk and half and half mix, simmer

(but do not boil), until hot. Season with salt and pepper, to taste. Add fresh parsley with 2 tablespoons of additional butter, to finish, if desired.
Nightshade free

CHICKEN TORTELLINI SOUP

Serves 4 main course servings.

1 ½ quarts chicken stock
1 ½ cups cooked chicken, diced
½ teaspoon garlic flakes (or 2 cloves, minced)
½ teaspoon black pepper
½ teaspoon salt
1 tablespoon dried parsley
(or 3 tablespoons fresh parsley, minced)
1 tablespoon preserved lemon, minced
(or 1-2 tablespoons lemon juice)
1 ½ cups tortellini
4 cups fresh spinach, loosely packed
1 cup mozzarella cheese, grated
½ cup half and half
1 tablespoon butter

Bring chicken stock to a boil, add cooked chicken, garlic, salt, pepper, parsley, and preserved lemon. Cook 5 minutes. Add tortellini and cook until tender, according to package directions. Add spinach, cook for 2 minutes, or until wilted. When ready to serve, add cheese, half and half, and butter. Adjust seasonings.
Nightshade free

GARLICKY KALE AND SWEET POTATO SOUP

My friend, Peggy, shared the following delicious and interesting soup recipe. Peggy, first told me about nightshades, and the harm they cause some people with arthritis. Her advice started my path to living an arthritis pain free life. Thank you, Peggy, for the advice and for the lovely soup. Serves 6.

2 tablespoons olive oil
1 large onion, chopped
4 teaspoons dried Italian herb mix
6 cups vegetable stock
2 - 15 oz. cans cannellini beans, rinsed and drained
1 lb. sweet potatoes, peeled and diced
4 cups kale, tough stems removed, coarsely chopped
12 garlic cloves, minced
Salt, pepper, and turmeric, to taste

In a large soup pot, saute onion in olive oil. Add the remaining ingredients, bring to a boil. Reduce to medium heat, simmer for 25-30 minutes, or until sweet potatoes are tender.

Nightshade free
Gluten free
Lactose free

SINGAPORE SPICY ASIAN SOUP

My friend Susan, who lives in Singapore, sent me a recipe for a spicy Asian soup that inspired this dish. The original recipe called for chipotle peppers in adobe sauce, that is replaced here with abundant white pepper which maintains the hot spicy, aromatic flavor. Use as much white pepper, as desired, without worry of nightshades. I've added additional vegetables and beans, which makes the soup hearty. This soup can be prepared vegetarian, or with chicken or shrimp, as desired. See directions below.
Preheat oven to 400 degrees. Serves 6.

1 acorn squash, sliced in 1 ½ in. wedges
1-2 tablespoons toasted sesame oil
(plus extra to brush acorn squash)
1 medium onion, chopped
4-5 garlic cloves, minced
2 quarts chicken stock
½ cup celery, sliced
2 cups mini carrots
2 cups frozen corn
2 cans white kidney beans (or cannellini), rinsed and drained
1 ½ cups raw diced chicken, optional
18-24 raw tiger shrimp (shell removed), optional
1-2 teaspoon white pepper, to taste
1 teaspoon black pepper
½ teaspoon salt
Juice of 1-2 limes, to taste
1 lime, cut in wedges (garnish)
1-2 avocados, sliced (garnish)
½ cup cilantro, chopped (garnish)
Corn tortillas

Carefully slice acorn squash into 1 ½ inch wedges. Brush with toasted sesame oil and place on a shallow baking dish. Roast for approximately 25-30 minutes, until tender. Cool slightly, remove skin from squash. Set aside. In a large soup pot, add 1-2 tablespoons toasted sesame oil, onion, and garlic. Sauté until golden brown. Add chicken stock, bring to boil. Then, simmer celery and carrots, until tender crisp. Return to boil, add corn, reduce heat and cook 3-5 minutes. Add beans, white and black peppers, salt, and lime juice. If adding raw chicken or shrimp, continue over medium high heat until chicken is done, or shrimp turns pink. Test seasoning, adding additional white pepper, to taste. Soup should be very spicy. Bring to a boil, add acorn squash and mix well. Top each serving with avocado slices, cilantro, and lime wedge. Serve with hot corn tortillas.

Nightshade free
Gluten free
Lactose free

THAI GINGER CHICKEN SOUP

My friend, Dasha, shared her recipe for this amazing Thai soup, which is a special Asian delight. Thai ginger adds heat and magic, without causing uncomfortable reactions from nightshades. Serves 4.

1 ½ cups chicken stock
3 cups unsweetened coconut milk (regular preferred)
1 inch section of Thai ginger, peeled and minced
3 tablespoons fish sauce
¼ cup fresh lime juice
3 tablespoons minced white onion
12.5 oz. can chicken breast, including broth
3-4 tablespoon fresh cilantro (garnish)
3-4 tablespoons green onions, sliced (garnish)

Combine chicken stock, coconut milk, ginger, fish sauce, lime juice, and white onion, in a medium pot. Bring to a boil, then reduce heat, and simmer 5-10 minutes. Add chicken with broth, simmer for 5 minutes. Serve hot, garnished with cilantro and green onions.

Nightshade free
Gluten free
Lactose free

PUREE OF SPLIT PEA AND VEGETABLE SOUP

Serves 6-8.

1 package green split peas, washed and picked over
2 quarts chicken stock
2 cups small carrots, coarsely chopped
1 medium onion, coarsely chopped
2-3 garlic cloves, minced
1 tablespoon dried oregano
Salt and pepper, to taste
2 tablespoons preserved lemon, minced
Water, as needed while cooking

Place green split peas and above ingredients, in a large soup pot. Bring to a boil, then reduce to simmer. Add water, if necessary. Cook for approximately 45-50 minutes, partially covered, or until peas are very tender. Add the following ingredients and proceed as follows:

3 cups cabbage, coarsely chopped
2 whole zucchini, sliced
Butter and fresh parsley

Add cabbage and zucchini, cook until tender. Slightly cool. Puree soup until smooth, using a stick blender, or use food processor. Add additional chicken stock, or water, for desired consistency. Reheat. Place hot servings in soup bowls, with a pat of butter and sprig of fresh parsley.

Nightshade free
Gluten free
Lactose free (omit butter garnish)

SOUTHWEST BUTTERNUT SQUASH SOUP

The spicy southwest flavors of this soup are created with thyme, cumin, white and black peppers. Make it as hot and spicy as you like, with additional white and black peppers, but without concern about nightshade discomfort.

Puree to a beautifully smooth, golden consistency. To roast butternut squash, preheat oven to 400 degrees. Serves 4-6.

2 lbs. butternut squash, cut in pieces (see below)
1 onion, chopped
2 ribs celery, chopped
3 cloves garlic, chopped
3 tablespoons olive oil
1 medium sweet potato, peeled and diced
1 apple, diced (do not peel)
4 cups chicken stock
1 cup water
1 heaping teaspoon thyme
1 heaping teaspoon cumin
Salt, white and black peppers, to taste
Light sour cream, garnish
Fresh parsley sprigs, garnish

To prepare butternut squash, carefully halve, remove seeds and membrane. Place on a baking dish. Roast for approximately 35-45 minutes, or until tender. Remove from oven and cool. Cut flesh from squash, in small pieces. Place onion, celery, garlic, and olive oil, in a large soup pot, caramelize ingredients. Add roasted squash, sweet potato, apple, chicken stock, water, thyme, cumin, salt, and peppers, to soup pot. Bring to a boil, cover and reduce heat to simmer. Cook 20-30 minutes. When vegetables are *soft*, cool slightly. Then, use stick blender or food processor, to puree soup. Reheat when ready to serve. Garnish with a dollop of light sour cream and sprig of parsley.

Nightshade free
Gluten free
Lactose free (omit sour cream garnish)

CARROT AND GINGER SOUP

Serves 6

6 tablespoons butter
1 large onion, chopped
¼ cup fresh Thai ginger, minced
3-4 garlic cloves, minced
7 cups chicken stock
1 cup dry white wine
2 lbs. carrots (chopped in food processor)
2 tablespoons fresh lemon juice
1-2 teaspoons curry powder (without cayenne and paprika)
Kosher salt and black pepper, to taste

In a large pot, melt butter. Add onion, ginger, and garlic. Saute about 10 minutes, over medium heat. Add chicken stock, wine, and carrots, bring to a boil. Partially cover and reduce heat to simmer. Cook about 30-35 minutes, or until carrots are soft. Add lemon juice, curry, salt and pepper. Cool slightly, puree with a stick blender or food processor. Adjust seasonings.

Nightshade free
Gluten free

CREAM OF CELERY AND HERB SOUP

I started making this soup back in the 1970s. It's changed over the years. There's no longer cream, and much less butter, but it's still a flavorful soup. Using a food processor to chop the vegetables, makes this soup a snap to prepare. Serves 4-6.

1-2 stalks celery (or 4-5 cups)
1 medium onion
5-6 garlic cloves
1 cup fresh parsley
½ cup butter

3 tablespoons flour
1% or 2 % milk (about 4-5 cups)
1 teaspoon ground sage
1 tablespoon Italian herb mix
1 teaspoon dried basil
Kosher salt, black and white peppers, to taste

Cut celery, onion, and garlic into chunky pieces. Coarsely chop fresh parsley. Add these ingredients to a food processor in batches, to further chop. Pulse works best for this method. Melt butter in a soup pot, then add vegetables. Add additional butter, if needed. When ingredients are very hot and sizzle, add flour and cook until a paste forms. Begin to add milk slowly, whisking constantly as soup develops. Add additional milk, if needed. When soup is preferred consistency, add dried herbs and seasonings. Blend well, bring to a light simmer, but do not boil. This soup is better, if chilled for a few hours, then reheated.

Nightshade free

SALADS FOR ALL SEASONS

SALADS FOR ALL SEASONS

Many foods we enjoy throughout the year focus on the seasons, and salad themes certainly vary according to what's available and freshest. Some of the selections below can stand alone as a main course, reflect a holiday or special occasion, while others are simple accompaniments to almost any meal.

Nightshades played a significant role in my traditional salads. In particular, I knew a worthy replacement for tomatoes would be difficult to find, and I was afraid that my salads would lose appeal and flavor. However, after taking a closer look at other colorful options, salads became not only interesting without nightshades, but satisfying. Try some of my favorite salad and dressing recipes, without nightshades. Many are gluten and lactose free, as well.

A SIMPLE FAVORITE

Serves 4.

Juice of ½ lemon
1/3 cup olive oil
Kosher salt and black pepper, to taste
3 cups arugula
2 cups red leaf lettuce, torn into pieces
½ cup Parmesan or feta cheese, or combination

Whisk lemon juice, olive oil, salt and pepper, set aside. In a large salad bowl, gently toss the greens with cheese. Add desired amount of salad dressing. Adjust seasonings, if necessary, and serve immediately.

Nightshade free
Gluten free
Lactose free (omit cheese)

WHITE WINE VINAIGRETTE

This delicate vinaigrette makes almost any salad sing! It's a version of *Champagne Vinaigrette,* found in this chapter. However, white wine vinegar is less expensive than champagne vinegar. For a slightly different flavor, try using fresh lime juice in this recipe. Dressing for 2 salads.

1 large garlic clove, minced
2 tablespoons Dijon mustard
¼ cup white wine vinegar
2 tablespoons fresh lemon or lime juice
1 ½ teaspoons agave, to taste (or substitute honey)
½ teaspoon salt
½ teaspoon black pepper
½ cup olive oil

Whisk first 7 ingredients. Then, whisk in olive oil, until emulsified.

Nightshade free
Gluten free
Lactose free

CAROLINE'S CAESAR SALAD

Over the years, I've changed this recipe a dozen times. When you marry anchovies, fresh lemon juice, yellow mustard, garlic, and Worcestershire, magic happens! If you like tangy, you may like this version of Caesar salad. Originally, I used a fork to mash the anchovy and garlic, but a small food processor works best, and you can blend all the ingredients at the same time. Over the years, I omitted the raw egg. Also, I do not recommend using my recipe, *Prune Enhanced Worcestershire Sauce,* for this dressing. A rich red wine, such as a Cabernet Sauvignon, Malbec, or Shiraz are excellent choices with this dish.

Serves 4

1 tin flat anchovies, drained slightly and minced
1/4 teaspoon Kosher salt
2 teaspoons black pepper, rounded
2 tablespoons yellow mustard, rounded
3/4 cup olive oil
1/3 cup fresh lemon juice
3 tablespoons Worcestershire Sauce (without chili extract)
6 cloves garlic, minced, or to taste
1 cup Parmesan cheese, grated
2-3 hearts of romaine lettuce, torn into bite size pieces
(or 1 1/2 large heads of romaine lettuce)
Croutons

In small food processor, add first 8 ingredients, blend until smooth. Toss dressing with romaine, Parmesan, and croutons, but be careful not to over-dress. Serve immediately, as lemon juice tends to wilt the lettuce.

Nightshade free
Gluten Free (omit croutons)

SIMPLE, SURPRISING SLAW

Cabbage slaw has been a staple in our family for years. But, this easy, delicious version brings a light, freshness to traditional slaw. Because it is so quick to make, and fresh is important with this recipe, I recommend preparing enough for one meal at a time. Serves 2-3.

½ large head green cabbage, coarsely chopped
½ cup Italian parsley, coarsely chopped
5-6 radishes, sliced
Salt and black pepper, to taste
Olive oil
White wine vinegar

Combine the cabbage, parsley, radishes, salt and pepper. Toss with desired amounts of olive oil and white wine vinegar. Serve immediately.
Nightshade free
Gluten free
Lactose free

ROASTED PEAR SALAD WITH ARUGULA

This elegant salad is a treat, comprised of simple ingredients, and presents beautifully. The roasted pears, can also be served as a dessert, with a ginger cranberry sauce, blueberry sauce, or fresh strawberries. Serves 4.

Preheat oven 375 degrees.
2 large ripe pears
¼ cup canola oil, plus ½ teaspoon agave, whisk together
2 cups arugula
½ cup goat cheese, softened
6-8 tablespoons toasted pecans
½ cup prosciutto

Halve pears, then remove core and veining. Brush with canola oil and agave mix, and place on a shallow baking dish (lined with foil, also lightly brushed with oil). Roast pears until golden and tender, approximately 20-30 minutes. Cooking time depends on ripeness of pears. Cool. On four individual serving plates, place pears on a small bed of arugula, add a few crumbles of goat cheese, a serving of pecans, and a curl of prosciutto.
Nightshade free
Gluten free
Lactose free (omit goat cheese)

CALICO SALAD

This is a special salad, my friend, Pat, in Oklahoma City, enjoys while sitting on her patio watching a sunset. The sunset and salad make a perfect ending to a busy day. Serves 3-4.

4-5 cups favorite greens
1- 1 ½ cups cauliflower, in small pieces
1 cup sharp cheddar cheese, small diced
2-3 hard boiled eggs, diced
¾ cup green onions, sliced
1 cup green olives, sliced (without pimento)
3-4 slices bacon, fried crisp and crumbled
Your favorite vinaigrette

Place all ingredients in a large salad bowl, except vinaigrette. When ready to serve, toss salad with a small amount of dressing. Note: Try *Champagne Vinaigrette,* or *Georgia O'Keeffe's Herb Salad Dressing,* recipes follow.

Nightshade free
Gluten free

GEORGIA O'KEEFFE'S HERB SALAD DRESSING

Being an abstract oil painter, I was delighted to discover Georgia O'Keeffe's cookbook and this delicious salad dressing. She had a love of gardening, and I like to imagine her picking herbs at Abiquiu in New Mexico, for this special dressing. Lovage is an old herb, used for good health, and is perfect for today's lifestyles. Lovage has a unique flavor, similar to anise and celery, and can be used as a salt substitute. Serving for 1-2 salads.

2 teaspoons mixed herbs, minced
(lovage, tarragon, dill, basil, and parsley)
2 tablespoons olive oil
2 tablespoons safflower oil

1 teaspoon fresh lemon juice, or to taste
¼ teaspoon whole mustard seed
2 cloves garlic, minced
Salt, to taste
Freshly ground black pepper
Pinch of sugar
Chives, for garnish

Whisk the ingredients to blend, and lightly dress very fresh greens. Garnish with chives, and think about Georgia!

Nightshade free
Gluten free
Lactose free

CHRISTMAS SALAD

Never pass up pomegranate season! To remove arils from pomegranate, slice in half, then remove carefully from membrane. Arils are the juice sacs, which is the essence of the fruit. Serves 8.

Large head red leaf lettuce, rinsed and dried
2 -3 cups spinach leaves, rinsed and dried
2 large grapefruits, peeled, cut in thin section slices
2 large avocados, in slices
1 pomegranate, arils removed and saved
¾ cup feta cheese, crumbled
½ cup pine nuts
¼ cup fresh lemon juice
3/4 cup olive oil
1 teaspoon oregano, dried
salt and pepper, to taste

Tear lettuce into bite size pieces, and arrange on a large platter mixed with spinach leaves. Place grapefruit sections in a circle around the lettuce, followed by the avocados, pomegranate arils (juice sacs), feta, and pine nuts. Prepare dressing by whisking lemon juice, olive oil, oregano, salt and pepper. When ready to serve, drizzle the dressing over the salad, but do not toss. Serve immediately. Serves 8.

Nightshade free
Gluten free
Lactose free (omit feta)

BERRY MIX SALAD

Serves 6.

1 -2 heads of red leaf lettuce
(rinsed, dried and torn into pieces)
1 English cucumber, thinly sliced
4-5 mushrooms, thinly sliced
1 ½ cups frozen berry mix, thaw and reserve juice
(such as raspberry, blackberry, blueberry mix)
½ cup feta cheese
Vinaigrette (recipe below)

Layer lettuce, cucumber, and mushrooms on a large platter or serving dish. When ready to serve, carefully layer the berries and about ½ cup of juice over the salad. Then add feta. Dress lightly with vinaigrette, as the juice from the berries becomes part of the dressing. For a beautiful presentation, toss at the table when served.

Simple vinaigrette:
1/2 cup olive oil
3 tablespoons red wine vinegar
1 teaspoon Dijon mustard
½ teaspoon oregano
salt and pepper, to taste

Nightshade free

Gluten free
Lactose free (omit feta cheese)

RED CABBAGE, APPLE, AND GREEN PEA LAYERED SALAD

A special layered salad is a lovely addition for any festive occasion. My friend, Jeanne, shares this one. Prepare this salad several hours in advance, or the night before serving. Serves 8 - 10.

2 cups frozen green peas, cooked, drained, and cooled
2 cups red cabbage, shredded
1 cup water chestnuts, drained
1/3 cup onion, chopped
3 green onions, sliced
1 cup celery, thinly sliced
1 large Granny Smith apple (or other favorite), unpeeled, cored, and diced
Kosher salt, to taste
½ cup light sour cream
½ cup mayonnaise
1 teaspoon sugar
1 cup cheddar cheese, grated
1 cup toasted pecans, finely chopped

At least 8 hours before serving, combine peas, cabbage, water chestnuts, onion, green onion, celery, apple, and salt, in a large bowl. Combine sour cream, mayonnaise, and sugar, mixing well. Spread the sour cream mixture over the cabbage mixture, covering the entire surface of the salad. Add a layer of the cheese, followed by a layer of pecans. Cover tightly and refrigerate. When ready to serve, gently toss to combine ingredients.

Nightshade free
Gluten free

RADICCHIO, PEAR, AND GORGONZOLA SALAD

Serves 4.

2 tablespoons olive oil
2 heads radicchio, rinsed and dried
2 tablespoons shallot, minced
1/3 cup pine nuts
1 large ripe pear, sliced
1/3 cup Gorgonzola cheese, crumbled
1/3 cup olive oil
3-4 tablespoons balsamic vinegar
Salt and pepper, to taste

In a medium skillet, add 2 tablespoons olive oil, and heat. Sear the radicchio leaves until slightly browned, transfer to paper towels to drain and cool. Add the shallot and pine nuts to the skillet, toss to sear the shallot and toast the nuts. On four salad plates, divide the seared radicchio, pear slices, shallot and pine nut mix, then top with Gorgonzola. Whisk olive oil, balsamic vinegar, salt and pepper, to taste. Drizzle over each salad.

Nightshade free

STRAWBERRY PRETZEL SALAD

Another wonderful salad from Oklahoma City, and my friend, Susan. This salad is perfect for any holiday gathering, but a delight anytime. Salad can be prepared 24 hours in advance, but no longer. Serves 8-10.

PRETZEL BASE Preheat oven to 400 degrees.
Pretzels, crushed to 2 cups textured crumbs
½ stick butter
½ cup sugar

Mix pretzel crumbs, butter, and sugar, then press in bottom of a 9x12 pan. Bake 8 minutes, then cool.

CREAM CHEESE FILLING
¼ cup sugar
8 oz. softened cream cheese
8 oz. Cool Whip

Blend sugar and cream cheese, until smooth, then fold in Cool Whip. Spread over pretzel crust base. Chill for 1-2 hours.

2 (3 oz.) packages strawberry or strawberry/banana Jello
10-12 oz. frozen strawberries, sliced

Prepare Jello as directed, and chill to slightly gel. Thaw strawberries only slightly, then fold into Jello. Pour over salad (pretzel crust and cream cheese filling), return to refrigerator to completely set, 2-3 hours. Do not freeze. When ready to serve, cut into squares, and place over a lettuce leaf on individual serving plates.

Nightshade free

CHAMPAGNE VINAIGRETTE

This special salad dressing is perfect on many salads, and turns simple mixed greens into something your guests will rave about. Serves 2 salads.

1 garlic clove, minced
2 tablespoons Dijon mustard
¼ cup champagne vinegar
2 tablespoons fresh lemon juice
1 ½ teaspoons agave, to taste (or substitute honey)
½ teaspoon salt
½ teaspoon black pepper
½ cup olive oil

Whisk first 7 ingredients, then whisk in olive oil, until emulsified.

Nightshade free
Gluten free
Lactose free

RED LEAF LETTUCE WITH CARROT AND WATERCRESS

This delicate salad is a winner with champagne vinaigrette (recipe above). Serves 4

1 head red leaf lettuce, rinsed, dried and torn into pieces
1 cup watercress, rinsed and dried
1 cup thin carrot strips (see note below)
6 radishes, thinly sliced
1/3 cup champagne vinaigrette (previous recipe)
2 miniature English cucumbers, thinly sliced
1/2 cup feta cheese
½ cup walnuts, toasted

Toss lettuce, watercress, carrot strips, and radishes with vinaigrette. Place on four salad plates. Pull some of the watercress and radish to the outer edges of lettuce. Arrange cucumbers around salads. Garnish each salad with feta cheese and walnuts. Note: To make thin carrot strips, firmly slide zester/stripper down sides of whole carrot, cutting long, thin strings that curl.

Nightshade free
Gluten free
Lactose free (omit feta cheese)

LARGE PARTY SALAD WITH ARTICHOKES

My daughter, Claire, gave me the original recipe for the Pasta House dinner salad, which is served in Pasta House Restaurants in St. Louis and Cape Girardeau, Missouri. I've adapted the recipe, omitting pimentos, which are nightshades, and added spinach. This is the perfect salad for large crowds, and is a hit every time it's served. Serves 8-12.

1 head iceberg lettuce, rinsed, dried and torn into pieces
1 ½ heads romaine lettuce, rinsed,
dried and torn into pieces

3 cups spinach leaves, rinsed and dried
1-2 cups oil packed artichokes, drained and chopped
1 cup red onion, thinly sliced
2/3 cup Parmesan cheese
Dressing:
2/3 cup olive oil
1/3 cup red wine vinegar
1 teaspoon salt
½ teaspoon black pepper

In a large salad bowl toss half the salad mixture (iceberg, romaine, spinach, artichokes, onion), half the Parmesan cheese, and half the dressing. Repeat steps in same salad bowl, blending with first mixture, tossing well. Let set approximately 30-45 minutes before serving. The salad wilts slightly, which is part of the essence.

Nightshade free
Gluten free

FAT FREE SPINACH SURPRISE SALAD

My friend, Coila, shares this wonderfully simple, but delicious salad. It's a great choice for casual suppers, holiday buffets, or a special treat at brunch. Serves 2.

10 oz. fresh spinach, rinsed and dried
2 tablespoons red onion, minced
2 tablespoons apple jelly
1/8 teaspoon salt
2 teaspoons cider vinegar

Place spinach and onion in a medium salad bowl. Microwave apple jelly on high for 30-45 seconds, or until melted. Add salt and cider vinegar to jelly, mix well. Toss with salad. Serves 2.

Nightshade free

Gluten free
Lactose free

CABERNET BUTTERMILK DRESSING

This smooth and delicious buttermilk dressing is a lovely substitute for traditional ranch dressing. Cabernet vinegar adds special flavor. See directions below for making buttermilk.

2 cups mayonnaise
1 cup buttermilk (see below)
3 tablespoons cabernet vinegar
3 teaspoons fresh parsley
3 teaspoons fresh thyme
3 teaspoons fresh basil
1 ½ tablespoons onion, minced
Kosher salt, white and black peppers, to taste

For buttermilk substitute: Add 1 tablespoon white vinegar or lemon juice to 1 cup regular milk, let stand 5 minutes. Combine all ingredients, whisk well, refrigerate for an hour.

Nightshade free
Gluten free

BLUE CHEESEBURGER SALAD

If you enjoy your hamburger wrapped in a lettuce leaf, then you'll love this salad. Recipe for 1.

½ pound 80-85% fat free organic hamburger meat, freshly ground
Salt and black pepper, to taste
½ teaspoon *each* garlic and onion powder

1/3 cup sweet onion, thinly sliced
1 teaspoon olive oil
2-3 radishes, thinly sliced (reserve 3 slices for garnish)
¼ cup dried cranberries
¼ cup toasted almonds, sliced
¼ cup carrots, minced
3 large lettuce leaves, torn in pieces
¼ cup champagne vinaigrette (recipe above)
(or commercial ranch dressing)
2 tablespoons blue cheese or Gorgonzola
Yellow or Dijon mustard

Preheat gas grill to 400-450 degrees. Press salt, pepper, garlic and onion powders, into both sides of hamburger patty. Use extra black pepper, as desired. Set aside. Microwave sweet onion and olive oil in a small dish, set aside. Combine radishes, cranberries, almonds, carrots, and lettuce with vinaigrette, and arrange on a large dinner plate. Grill burger, as preferred. When nearly done, add cheese to one side of burger, close grill lid for 1-2 minutes to melt. Place burger in center of salad, topped with hot onions. Garnish with radish slices and side of mustard.

Nightshade free
Gluten free
Lactose free (omit cheese)

Note: Yellow mustards may contain paprika, which can cause problems for some individuals.

CAROLINE'S SALAD NICOISE

This is an amazing entrée for summer dinner parties, fun for the cook, and fun for the guests. I arrange everything on a *mega size* platter, then place in the middle of the dining table on a tea towel, folded square. This protects the table, and helps the platter turn easily for guests to serve themselves. There are many grand versions of this classic salad, but this one has no nightshades. I use Aji/sushi grade tuna steaks, seared rare, as the focal point of the platter. Canned tuna in oil is the French traditional choice in many recipes, which can replace the tuna steaks, if you choose. Even though there are several steps to complete this salad, everything can be prepared hours before serving, freeing the hostess of last-minute preparation. Serves 8.

VINAIGRETTE

½ cup fresh lemon juice, plus 2-3 tablespoons
1 cup olive oil
1 medium shallot, minced
2 tablespoon fresh thyme leaves, minced
4 tablespoons fresh basil leaves, minced
2 teaspoons fresh oregano leaves, minced
1 teaspoon Dijon mustard
Salt and black pepper

Whisk above ingredients and refrigerate.

SALAD

16 oz. Aji/sushi grade tuna steaks
Olive oil
10 hard boiled eggs
1-2 tablespoons Dijon mustard
1/3 cup mayonnaise
1 tablespoon sweet pickle relish (without red peppers)
Salt and white pepper
1 red onion, thinly sliced
1 ½ cup oil packed artichoke hearts
24 fresh asparagus spears
4-5 slices bacon, fried crisp and crumbled
1 large English cucumber, peeled and sliced
10 radishes, cut in rosettes

1 ½ - 2 heads red leaf lettuce,
rinsed, dried, and torn in large pieces
2 large ripe avocados, sliced
1/2 cup capers, drained
¾ cup Kalamata olives, pitted
1-2 tins anchovies, drained

Marinate (and refrigerate) tuna steaks for at least 1 hour in olive oil, salt and pepper. Remove from refrigerator, 15 minutes before grilling (or to sear, in hot iron skillet on stove). Sear fish rare, or as desired. Slice into 8 pieces and drizzle 3 tablespoons of vinaigrette on the fish, turn pieces to coat. Return to refrigerator.

Boil the eggs, peel, and slice in half. Remove yokes and place in a small bowl. Add Dijon mustard, mayonnaise, and sweet relish, mashing with fork until smooth. For a fluffier filling, add additional mayonnaise. Season with salt and white pepper. Stuff egg whites with yoke mixture, refrigerate.

Toss red onion and artichoke hearts, with 2 tablespoons vinaigrette, place in container and refrigerate. Steam the asparagus slightly, place in a ice water bath. Drain and pat dry. Place in separate container, drizzle 3 tablespoons of vinaigrette over the asparagus, refrigerate. Fry bacon, crumble and set aside.

Prep cucumbers, radishes, lettuce, and refrigerate. Prep avocados, just before serving. Arrange capers, olives, and anchovies on salad, as platter it assembled.

When ready to serve, arrange lettuce on the platter, place tuna in center. Lattice anchovies over fish, or to one side. Arrange other components of the salad around the tuna, in groups. Drizzle 1/3 cup vinaigrette, over the salad (except the deviled eggs), then sprinkle the crumbled bacon. Serve immediately. Pass additional vinaigrette at the table.

Nightshade free
Gluten free
Lactose free

SOUTHERN (SWEET) POTATO SALAD

Potato salad has been a staple at summer barbeques, picnics, and reunions, in our family for decades. But, without white potatoes? Check this out.
Serves 6-8.

3 cups cooked sweet potatoes, peeled and sliced
(salt and pepper, while cooking)
1 cup celery, minced
½ cup white onion, minced
½ cup mayonnaise
2 heaping tablespoons Dijon mustard
3 hard boiled eggs, diced
¼ cup sweet relish (without red peppers)
1/8 cup fresh lemon juice, or to taste
Kosher salt and black pepper, to taste

Bring potatoes to a boil, cover slightly, and simmer until tender. Drain well, and mix with remaining ingredients, while potatoes are warm.

Nightshade free
Gluten free
Lactose free

FISH AND SEAFOOD TO DELIGHT

FISH AND SEAFOOD TO DELIGHT

Cooking with fish or seafood is versatile and easy. Pairing these entrée choices with pasta or grains, vegetables, sauces, or in soups, makes an exciting meal for yourself and your guests.

ASIAN SHRIMP TACOS

2 Servings

2 whole wheat tortillas
1 ½ cup red cabbage, finely sliced
½ cup onion, diced
4-5 mushrooms, sliced
2-4 tablespoons olive oil
2 garlic cloves, minced
1 teaspoon dried ground ginger
(or 1 tablespoon fresh ginger, minced)
Salt and white pepper
6-8 raw medium shrimp, peeled
2-3 tablespoons tamari, to taste
¾ cup sugar snap peas
Sesame Soy Sauce (found in oriental section of grocery)
1/3 cup fresh basil, coarsely chopped (garnish)

Place one tortilla on each serving plate, with a layer of cabbage. Sauté onion and mushrooms, in olive oil. Add garlic, ginger, salt and pepper, mixing well. To hot vegetable/seasoning mixture, add shrimp, with 2-3 tablespoons tamari, tossing 3-4 minutes over medium high heat, or until shrimp is pink. Additional olive oil may be required. Add sugar snap peas to shrimp and vegetables, mix well. Cover to steam for 2 minutes. Adjust seasonings. Place

shrimp/vegetable mixture on top of the tortilla and cabbage, followed by 3 tablespoons of Sesame Soy Sauce (or other favorite oriental sauce). Garnish with fresh basil. Pass additional Sesame Soy Sauce and tamari, at table.
Nightshade free
Lactose free

STEAMED WILD SALMON WITH MUSTARD GREENS, TAMARI, AND GINGER

This flavorful wild salmon recipe (*Relish Magazine, 2011),* was discovered and originally prepared, by my friend, Jeanne. Her version of this recipe is nightshade, gluten, and lactose free. Farm raised salmon can be substituted for wild salmon, if you choose. Serves 4.

1 tablespoon vegetable oil
1 teaspoon toasted sesame oil (plus additional for drizzle)
3 cloves garlic, minced
1 inch slice fresh ginger, peeled and minced
1 pound mustard greens or kale, carefully washed (stems removed and torn into pieces)
1-2 tablespoon tamari
Water
2 - 6-8 oz. wild salmon filets
Kosher salt and coarse black pepper, to taste

Heat oils in a very large skillet, with lid. Add garlic and ginger, saute until fragrant. Spread greens, tamari, and 1/3 cup water in bottom of skillet (over garlic and ginger), cover and steam for 2 minutes. Top with fish, salt and pepper. (If evaporated, add 2-4 tablespoons additional water.) Cover again, reduce heat to medium. Steam fish to medium or medium-well, about 4-8 minutes, as desired. Place fish, over a serving of the greens, with a drizzle of additional sesame oil and tamari. Serve immediately.

Nightshade free
Gluten free
Lactose free

RUBY RED TROUT ON THE GRILL WITH LIME

This simple, but elegant approach to preparing ruby red trout is a healthy, low calorie, and delicious way to enjoy this special fish. Preheat gas grill to 450 degrees. Serves 4.

4 ruby red trout filets, rinsed and dried
Vegetable oil spray
2 limes, cut in wedges
Kosher salt and pepper, to taste
1-2 teaspoons dill weed
2-3 tablespoons butter

Make 4 small *foil boats* to hold individual filets, by crimping corners of foil. Place boats on a cookie sheet that can be used on the grill. Coat foil with vegetable oil spray. Add fish. Squeeze lime juice over each filet, season with salt, pepper, and dill weed. Add 3-4 dots of butter to each fish. Place on gas grill for 5-6 minutes, covered. Serve, with lime wedges.

Nightshade free
Gluten free

SALMON CAKES

Serves 4.

2 6 oz. cans boneless/skinless salmon, drained
2 eggs
½ cup mushrooms, minced
1/3 cup carrot, minced

½ cup celery, minced
¼ cup onion, minced
½ cup Italian bread crumbs
Salt and pepper, to taste
1 teaspoon dried basil
1 tablespoon dried parsley
1 tablespoon fresh lemon juice
Olive oil
Lemon or lime wedges, garnishes

Toss, first 11 ingredients gently, careful not to over mix. Refrigerator for 30-45 minutes. Heat a large skillet prepared with a thin layer of olive oil. Avoid over heating or smoking. Form salmon cakes into patties, about 1 ½ inches in diameter. Place patties in hot skillet, pan fry for 2-3 minutes, or until golden brown. Turn once, and cook an additional 2-3 minutes. Serve immediately, with lemon or lime wedges.

Nightshade free
Lactose free

MUSSELS WITH WHITE WINE AND HERBS

Serves 2-4.

40-50 fresh mussels
2 cups white wine
2-3 cups chicken stock, as needed
½ cup shallots, minced
4 garlic cloves, minced
3 tablespoons butter
1 teaspoon (each) dried thyme and oregano
1-2 bay leaves
1 teaspoon white pepper, or taste

Kosher salt, to taste
Crusty bread and butter (at table)

Keep mussels on ice in refrigerator, until ready to steam. Wash under cold running water, removing *beard,* grit, etc. Sort and discard any mussels that are not firmly closed, or those that do not close when tapped. Keep mussels in ice water bath, until stock mixture is prepared. In a large stock pot, add wine, chicken stock, shallots, garlic, 3 tablespoons butter, herbs, bay leaf, white pepper, and salt. Bring to a rolling boil, add mussels. Cover and return to boil. Mussels cook quickly, usually in minutes, but are done when they open and are plump. DO NOT SERVE MUSSELS THAT HAVE NOT OPENED. Remove mussels immediately with a slotted spoon, trying not to disturb any sediment in bottom of pot. Arrange mussels in individual serving bowls, with ample stock/wine mixture. Serve with crusty bread and butter, for dipping in broth.

Nightshade free
Gluten free (use gluten free bread)
Lactose free (omit butter)

SALMON IN CORNMEAL CRUST OVER ARUGULA

Serves 2

1 egg
½ cup milk
½ teaspoon garlic flakes (or 1 large garlic clove, minced)
Salt and coarse black pepper, to taste
1 tablespoon dehydrated onion
2 salmon filets
¾ cup cornmeal
1 tablespoon dried parsley flakes

1 teaspoon black pepper
Olive oil
3-4 cups arugula, rinsed and dried
1-2 tablespoons fresh lemon or lime juice
Lemon or lime wedges, garnishes

Whisk egg, milk, garlic, salt, pepper, and dehydrated onion. Pour over salmon filets. Refrigerate for approximately 1 hour. Set out 15 minutes prior to cooking. In a shallow dish, mix cornmeal, with parsley flakes and black pepper, set aside. In a medium skillet, cover bottom with ½ inch olive oil. As oil heats to medium high, remove salmon from egg mix, dredge all sides in cornmeal mixture. In hot oil, pan sear filets on each side for 3-4 minutes, depending on thickness and desired doneness. Lay on paper towel, to drain. Toss arugula with lemon or lime juice and 3-4 tablespoons olive oil, salt and pepper. On serving plates, add a bed of arugula salad, top with the salmon filets. Serve with lemon or lime wedges.

Nightshade free
Gluten free

SHRIMP WITH ROSEMARY GARLIC PASTA

Serves 2

8-12 raw shrimp, depending on size
½ cup olive oil
1 teaspoon garlic flakes (or 1 large garlic clove, minced)
1 teaspoon dried basil
1 teaspoon dried oregano, or Italian herb mix
1 teaspoon dill weed
Salt and pepper, to taste
Juice of ½ lemon
½ small onion, minced
1 ½ ribs celery, minced

½ cup red wine
½ package curly pasta
(rosemary garlic flavoring, suggested)
½ cup cilantro, chopped (garnish)
Lemon or lime wedges (garnish)

Marinate shrimp in olive oil, garlic, basil, oregano, dill weed, salt, pepper, and lemon juice, for 45 minutes in refrigerator. Set out 15 minutes prior to cooking. Prepare pasta according to package directions, drain well. Pour shrimp mixture, onion, and celery, into preheated skillet, saute for 2-3 minutes. When shrimp turn pink, add ½ cup red wine, simmer 2 minutes. Remove from heat. If moisture is needed, add an additional 1-2 tablespoons olive oil. Place a serving of pasta on each plate, top with shrimp mixture. Garnish with cilantro, lemon or lime wedges.

Nightshade free
Gluten free
Lactose free

STEELHEAD TROUT OVEN ROASTED

This dish makes a lovely appetizer, served with gluten free crackers and herbed cream cheese, or as a main course. Preheat oven 400 degrees. Serves 4-6 as main course.

Vegetable oil spray
1 ½ - 2 lbs steelhead trout filet, rinsed and dried
Juice of ½ fresh lemon
2-3 tablespoons preserved lemon, minced
Black pepper, to taste
White pepper and salt, to taste
1 teaspoon dried oregano
Drizzle of olive oil

Prepare *boat* by turning up foil edges and crimping corners, allowing approximately 1 inch around sides of fish. Place foil boat on cookie sheet. Coat with vegetable oil spray, place trout on foil. Squeeze lemon juice over the fish, followed by preserved lemon, and seasonings. Drizzle 2 tablespoons olive oil, over fish. Place cookie sheet on middle rack of oven, roast for 15-18 minutes, depending on size. Be careful not to overcook.
Nightshade free
Gluten free
Lactose free

STEELHEAD TROUT IN PARMESAN CRUST

Preheat oven 425 degrees. Serves 4-6

Vegetable oil spray
Large steelhead trout filet
Juice of one lemon
Salt and black pepper, to taste
½ teaspoon garlic flakes (or 1 large garlic clove)
1 teaspoon dill weed, or 2 tablespoons fresh dill
Parmesan cheese
Butter

On a large cookie sheet, place a layer of foil, pinching corners to form a *boat.* Coat with vegetable oil spray, lay fish in center, tucking under the small end of fish. Slowly squeeze lemon juice over fish, to thoroughly coat. Sprinkle with salt, pepper, garlic flakes, and dill weed. Layer and press a heavy coating of Parmesan over fish. Top with several teaspoons of butter. Roast in oven for approximately 15-17 minutes, or until fish is medium to medium-well. Let stand, uncovered for 10 minutes before serving.
Nightshade free
Gluten free

STEELHEAD TROUT OR SALMON WITH CAROLINE'S DRY SPICY RUB

Preheat oven or gas grill to 400 degrees.

For something different, try *Caroline's Dry Spicy Rub* on steelhead trout or salmon. Simply press desired amount of rub on fish, refrigerate 1-2 hours. The more rub used, the spicier the fish. Set out 15 minutes prior to cooking. If a delicate crust is desired for the fish, drizzle lightly with olive oil before cooking. Roast in preheated oven, about 16-18 minutes. If you choose, place fish in double *foil boat*, and roast in preheated gas grill. Let stand 10 minutes before serving. Serve with fresh lime wedges. Serves 4-6 as main course.

Note: Recipe for *Caroline's Dry Spicy Rub* is found in *Beverages, Sauces, and Other Fun Stuff.*

Nightshade free

Gluten free

Lactose free

CAROLINE'S SALAD NICOISE

For this fish/salad entrée, and a delightful summer's evening with friends, see chapter: *Salads for All Seasons.*

PAN SEARED SCALLOPS WITH BLACK FORBIDDEN RICE

Serves 4

Black Forbidden Rice, cooked and well seasoned
12 large scallops, rinsed and dried
Salt and white pepper, to taste
3 tablespoons olive oil
1 medium shallot, minced

Juice of ½ lemon
½ cup white wine
Black truffle oil

Prepare black rice, season well, set aside. Salt and pepper the scallops, set aside. In a large skillet with olive oil, saute shallot, push to side of pan. Add scallops, at medium high heat, sear each side 2 minutes. Scallops should slightly brown and crisp. Be careful not to overcook. Remove scallops, cover with a tea towel to keep warm. Deglaze pan, on high heat, with lemon juice and ½ cup white wine, scraping all sides of pan. Reduce liquid to a thin syrup, adjust seasonings. To serve, place ½ cup black rice on plate, followed with serving of scallops. Drizzle reduction over shrimp, followed with a few drops of truffle oil, to finish. Serve immediately.

Nightshade free
Gluten free
Lactose free

RUBY RED TROUT WITH CORNMEAL AND PARSLEY CRUST

Serves 2. Three easy steps follow.

EGG WASH FOR FILETS
1 egg (for lighter crust, omit egg)
½ cup milk
2 ruby red trout filets
Salt and black pepper, to taste
½ teaspoon garlic flakes

Whisk egg and milk, pour over trout filets in a shallow bowl. Coat fish well. Sprinkle seasoning on filets. Refrigerate one hour. Set out 15 minutes before frying.

CORNMEAL MIXTURE
1 cup cornmeal

1 tablespoon dried parsley
½ teaspoon garlic flakes
1 teaspoon salt
1 teaspoon black pepper

Mix dry ingredients thoroughly, in a shallow dish.

PAN FRYING FILETS
Olive oil
Dill weed
Lemon and/or lime, garnish

Preheat large skillet with 1/2 inch olive oil. Oil should be hot, but not smoking. Turn filets to coat in egg wash, dip fish in cornmeal mixture, covering both sides. Place filets in hot skillet with oil, cook each side approximately 2 minutes. When done, lay on paper towels, sprinkle with dill weed. Serve with lemon and/or lime wedges.

Nightshade free
Gluten free

SHRIMP TOWERS WITH SWISS CHARD AND DILL

Serves 4

1 recipe of Cheese Grits, prepared and set aside (see *Savory Pastas and Grains*)
8 cups Swiss chard, tough stems removed and sliced
3-5 tablespoons olive oil
½ cup onion, chopped
2 garlic cloves, minced
1 rib celery, chopped
1 teaspoon salt
1 teaspoon white pepper
1 teaspoon black pepper
2 teaspoon dill weed

14-16 large tiger shrimp, peeled
1 cup dry or sweet vermouth, or white wine, as preferred

Cook cheese grits according to recipe found in *Savory Pastas and Grains,* set aside and keep warm. Wash and dry Swiss Chard, removing any tough stems, place in large skillet with 1-2 tablespoons water, cover and steam. Set aside. (If liquid remains, absorb with paper towel.) In a medium skillet, add 3-4 tablespoons olive oil, onion, garlic, celery, salt, peppers, and dill weed. Saute and bring to high heat. When mixture sizzles, add shrimp, tossing to coat and sauté, 1-2 minutes. Add vermouth or wine, mixing well. Cover for 1-2 minutes, or until shrimp is bright pink. Adjust seasonings.

To assemble:

On four dinner plates: Place a serving of cheese grits in center of each plate, spread to form a circle. Add a serving of Swiss Chard. Arrange 3-4 shrimp on each *tower,* followed by 3-4 tablespoons of sauce. Serve immediately.

Nightshade free
Lactose free (omit cheese from grits)
Gluten Free

SHRIMP OR SEA SCALLOP TOWERS WITH VERMOUTH AND GOAT CHEESE

This *tower recipe* can be prepared with shrimp or sea scallops. Each makes a perfect topping. However, the grand finale is the sauce, which is mellowed with a dollop of goat cheese. Serves 4.

1 recipe Cheese Grits, prepared and set aside
(see *Savory Pastas and Grains*)
8 cups spinach
4-5 tablespoons olive oil
1 teaspoon salt
1-2 teaspoon white pepper
1 teaspoon black pepper

2 teaspoon tarragon
3 garlic cloves, minced
½ cup onion, chopped
2 ribs celery, chopped
Juice of ½ lemon
14-16 large tiger shrimp
1 cup dry or sweet vermouth, or white wine, as preferred
2 tablespoons goat cheese, softened

Prepare Cheese Grits, according to directions found in *Savory Pastas and Grains.* Goat cheese is suggested, for this particular recipe of cheese grits. Set aside. Place spinach in a large skillet, with 2 tablespoons water, cover to steam, set aside. In a medium skillet, add olive oil, seasonings, tarragon, garlic, onion, celery, and lemon juice. Saute for 3-4 minutes. Push mixture to side of skillet, evenly layer shrimp (or scallops), in pan. Sear both sides, over medium high heat, for 1-2 minutes. Pour vermouth or wine over seafood. When vermouth is hot and steamy, add 2 tablespoons goat cheese, mixing all ingredients well, cover for 2 minutes. To Assemble: On four dinner plates, add a serving of Cheese Grits, forming a circle. Top with steamed spinach. Add 3-4 shrimp (or scallops) in center of tower, followed by serving of sauce.

Nightshade free
Gluten free

BACON WRAPPED SEA SCALLOPS WITH LIGHT BECHAMEL SAUCE

My friend, Marysia, selects this lovely scallops recipe for special occasions. The dish is delicate, the presentation memorable, and the flavors are amazing.

Preheat oven to 400 degrees, or broiler on high.

Serves 5-6.

1 package bacon strips
10-12 large sea scallops (2 per person)

3-5 tablespoons butter
2 teaspoons olive oil, optional
Toothpicks
Vegetable oil spray
3-4 tablespoons flour (for desired thickening)
½-1 cup 2% milk or half and half (or mix)
1 cup chicken stock (or more as needed)
1-2 teaspoons Kosher salt
White and black pepper, to taste
1/3- ½ cup Madeira sherry (optional)

In an iron skillet, or heavy pan, fry bacon until slightly browned, in 2 teaspoons of butter or olive oil. Bacon should be flexible (not crisp, for wrapping scallops). Remove bacon to cool. In same pan, quickly sear scallops, about 1 minute on each side. Place scallops and bacon on a work surface, gently wrap each scallop in one slice of bacon. Secure with toothpicks. Line a shallow baking pan with foil, coated with vegetable oil spray. Place scallops in pan, bake or broil in preheated oven, for approximately 4-8 minutes, or until done. Scallops should be lightly browned, but not overdone. If broiling, turn scallops after 2 minutes. While scallops are cooking in oven, prepare béchamel sauce by adding 3-4 additional tablespoons butter to same skillet, melt, and add flour, one tablespoon at a time, as desired for amount of sauce and thickening. When flour and butter form a soft paste, add 2% milk (or half and half), whisking continuously. Add chicken stock, as needed. When sauce is smooth and luscious, add seasonings and Madeira sherry, blending well.

To serve, place ¼ cup béchamel sauce in center of each serving plate, add scallops with bacon. Spoon a portion of sauce over scallops. Serve immediately.

Nightshade free
Gluten free

TILAPIA WITH CAPER RELISH

This simple fish gets dressed-up, when served with caper relish. The easy steps follow. Serves 4

RELISH
3 tablespoons olive oil, as needed
2 ribs celery, minced
1 large carrot, thinly sliced
1 cup onion, coarsely chopped
½ teaspoon garlic flakes
3-4 tablespoons capers
¼ cup fresh lemon juice, or 2 tablespoons preserved lemon
1-2 tablespoons dried parsley
2 teaspoons oregano
Salt and pepper, to taste

In a small skillet, saute celery, carrot, and onion in olive oil. Add remaining ingredients. Cook at medium heat for 4-5 minutes. Relish should be moist and chunky. Set aside. (Can be served room temperature or warm.)

MILK BATH
4 pieces tilapia, halved
1 cup milk
Salt and pepper, to taste
½ teaspoon garlic flakes

Mix milk with salt, pepper, and garlic flakes. Pour over tilapia.

CORNMEAL MIX
1 ½ cups cornmeal
½ teaspoon garlic flakes
2 tablespoon dried parsley
Salt and pepper, to taste
Olive oil

When ready to pan fry fish, heat ½ inch olive oil in a large skillet. Remove tilapia from milk mixture, roll in cornmeal mix. Pan fry in hot oil, turning once. Cook 2-3 minutes each side, according to thickness, or until golden brown. When ready to serve, place tilapia on a plate and garnish with approximately 1/3 cup caper relish.

Nightshade free

Gluten free

SCALLOPS WITH ALMONDS, TRUFFLE OIL, AND VEGETABLE COMPOTE

Serves 2

VEGETABLE COMPOTE

3 tablespoons olive oil

2 cups coarsely shredded cabbage

½ cup onion, thinly sliced

5 mushrooms, sliced

1 tablespoon dried parsley

1/2 teaspoon turmeric

½ teaspoon garlic flakes

2 tablespoons fresh lemon juice

¾ cup chicken stock

4 cups fresh spinach

Salt and pepper, to taste

Lightly saute first 9 ingredients, careful not to over cook. Add spinach, saute until slightly wilted. Season with salt and pepper, to taste. Set aside. Compote should resemble a chunky stew.

SCALLOPS, ALMONDS, TRUFFLE OIL

2-3 large scallops, per person

Salt and pepper, to taste

2-3 tablespoons olive oil

4 tablespoons slivered almonds, toasted (garnish)

Truffle oil

Season scallops with salt and pepper, coat in olive oil. Heat a dry, heavy skillet to medium-high heat, pan sear scallops 2 minutes on each side. Remove from heat.

ASSEMBLE

In two large, shallow soup bowls, add warm vegetable compote, topped with the seared scallops. Sprinkle with toasted almonds, to garnish. To finish, drizzle a bit of truffle oil over scallops. Serve immediately.

Nightshade free
Gluten free
Lactose free

SALMON EN PAPPITTOTE

Serves 6, as main course, or 12 as appetizer.
Preheat oven 425 degrees.

1 large, whole salmon filet
½ cup white wine
1 lime, juiced
Kosher salt and white pepper, to taste
½ cup fresh basil, chopped
2-4 garlic cloves, minced
¼ cup black olives, sliced
¼ cup Kalamata olives, halved
1 tablespoon capers
1/3 cup almond slivers
6-7 small pats of butter

Rinse and dry salmon, place on parchment paper (over a cookie sheet, with parchment large enough to enclose fish and seal). Pour wine and lime juice over salmon. Sprinkle with salt and pepper, followed by basil, garlic, both olives, capers, and almonds. Arrange pats of butter down center of fish. Fold parchment together to form a pouch, seal by folding over securely, or staple,

if necessary. (If using staples, be careful to remove before serving.) Bake in preheated oven for approximately 18-20 minutes, or as desired. When done, carefully slide the pouch with salmon, onto a large serving platter. Present at table or buffet *en pappittote,* before opening.
Nightshade free
Gluten free

SOUTHERN FRIED CATFISH WITH TARTER SAUCE AND LEMON WEDGES

When you've eaten really fresh, and really good fried catfish, there's nothing that will take it's place. Fresh is important, and may be difficult to find, outside the south. Tarter sauce is traditionally served with this dish, but fresh lemon juice is my choice. Serves 6.

8-10 large pieces fresh catfish
Kosher salt and black pepper, to taste
1 ½ quarts peanut or canola oil
2 eggs, beaten
2 cups milk
3 cups yellow corn meal
3 tablespoons dried parsley
1 teaspoon garlic flakes
Lemon wedges, garnish

Rinse and dry catfish, season with salt and pepper, to taste. Slowly heat about 2 ½ inches of oil, in a deep, heavy pan, on medium-high. An iron skillet is suggested. While oil is heating, mix milk and egg, set aside. Blend cornmeal, parsley, garlic flakes, and salt and pepper, set aside. Oil is ready for frying, when a sprinkle of cornmeal sizzles in the fat. (Very hot oil is necessary for flaky fish, with a crisp crust.) When oil is ready, dip one piece of fish in egg wash, then roll in cornmeal mixture. Gently drop one piece into hot oil. Follow with another piece, or two, depending on the size of pan, but do not crowd. Turn fish, when bottom side is very crisp. Fish will cook quickly (3-4 minutes), and is done when golden brown. Remove each piece carefully, and place on paper towels. Continue the process until all fish is cooked. Serve with tarter sauce (recipe below) and lemon wedges.

TARTER SAUCE

1 ½ cup mayonnaise
3/4 cup onion, minced
1 tablespoon lemon zest
2 tablespoons fresh lemon juice
2 tablespoons sweet relish (without red peppers)

Mix the ingredients above, chill. Serve with hot fish.

Nightshade free
Gluten free

CHICKEN WITH ZEST

CHICKEN WITH ZEST

Chicken is easy to prepare, a staple in most kitchens, and there are thousands of delicious, interesting recipes available everywhere. However, the following chicken recipes have no nightshades or seasonings derived from the nightshade plant family. Some are also gluten and lactose free, where indicated.

MOROCCAN CHICKEN WITH GREEN OLIVES AND LEMON

This chicken stew is a favorite for parties and fun evenings, with friends or family. For presentation, place cooked chicken on a platter with sauce, lemons, and olives. Serve additional sauce, at table. Or, serve chicken pieces in individual large soup bowls, with a serving of the sauce, etc. *Quinoa with Apricots and Golden Raisins,* is suggested as a side-dish, and is found in *Savory Pastas and Grains.* Serves 8-10.

2-3 large lemons
2-3 tablespoons olive oil
2 large onions, halved, then sliced
Salt and pepper, to taste
4 cloves garlic, minced
1 teaspoon turmeric
4 teaspoons ground cumin
2 teaspoons ground cinnamon
2 teaspoon ground ginger
4 cups chicken stock
10-14 assorted pieces of chicken
(halve breasts, to better absorb juice and flavors)
1 ½ -2 cups green olives stuffed with garlic

Cut lemons in wedges, and squeeze 4 tablespoons juice, to reserve. Set aside. In a large pan or stock pot, add olive oil and onions, with salt and pepper. Saute until slightly golden. Add garlic, turmeric, cumin, cinnamon, and ginger. Cook 1-2 minutes, adding olive oil, if needed. Add chicken stock, and bring to boil. Salt and pepper chicken pieces, add to boiling broth mixture, with lemon wedges and olives. Mix well, coating all chicken pieces in sauce. Cover, cook on high simmer, for approximately 25-30 minutes. Add reserved lemon juice, for increased lemon flavor, if desired. Stir several times, during cooking process. Serving suggestions above.

Nightshade free
Gluten free
Lactose free

GRILLED CHICKEN BREAST ON THE GRILL

Preheat gas grill to 450-475 degrees. Serves 6.

6 boneless/ skinless chicken breasts
1/3 cup olive oil
1 teaspoon salt
1 teaspoon black pepper
1 teaspoon white pepper
3 tablespoons Worcestershire sauce (without chili extract)
2 tablespoons lemon juice
2 tablespoons tamari
1 teaspoon garlic flakes (or 3 garlic cloves, minced)
1 tablespoon red wine vinegar
1 tablespoon onion, minced

Mix last 10 ingredients in a small bowl, pour over chicken in a large container. Coat chicken well, and refrigerate for 1 hour. Set out for 15 minutes, prior to cooking. When ready to cook, grill for approximately 6 minutes, on each side. Chicken will be crisp and brown on the outside, and juicy and tender inside. High temperature is key to this dish. Note: For an alternative to the marinade above, try Caroline's Dry Spicy Rub, found in *Beverages, Sauces, and Other Fun Stuff.*

Nightshade free
Gluten free
Lactose free

GRANNY SMITH CHICKEN TENDERS

The magic to this recipe is the sauce, which becomes a brilliant, dark red reduction that is rich in flavor. If doubling the recipe, be sure to double the sauce. Serves 3.

6-7 tablespoons butter, in total
1 large Granny Smith apple, unpeeled and diced
1 teaspoon honey or agave
1 teaspoon fresh lemon juice
1 cup flour
Salt and black pepper, to taste
10 chicken tenders
1 cup chicken stock
1 cup apple juice
½ cup cranberry juice
¼ -1/3 cup Madeira Sherry
Cinnamon stick
Sprigs of parsley, to garnish

Place 2 tablespoons butter in a small skillet. Add apple, honey or agave, and lemon juice. Sauté until apple is tender and slightly golden, 3-5 minutes. Set aside. Place flour in a bowl. Season chicken with salt and pepper, to taste, dredge chicken in flour. Have a large skillet heating over medium high heat, with 3-4 tablespoons butter, or more if needed. When butter sizzles, pan sear chicken tenders, for approximately 3-4 minutes, on each side, or until golden crisp. Remove to a plate, lined with paper towels. Cover loosely with foil, to keep warm. In same large skillet, add chicken broth, fruit juices, Madeira, and cinnamon stick. Bring to boil, scraping sides and bottom of pan, to release frying residue. Boil to reduce to 2/3-3/4 cup, approximately 15 minutes. Stir and scrape often. When reduction is finished, remove cinnamon stick and add 2-3 tablespoons butter. Stir in apple mixture, coating all pieces. Place chicken tenders on a serving platter, pour reduction and apples over chicken. Garnish with parsley sprigs.

Nightshade free

PESTO POCKET CHICKEN

Serves 2 Preheat oven to 400 degrees

2 boneless/skinless chicken breasts
2 tablespoon basil pesto
2 tablespoon pine nuts
4 tablespoons Parmesan cheese
Drizzle olive oil
Salt and pepper, to taste
Vegetable oil spray

Carefully cut a pocket in one side of each chicken breast. Season with salt and pepper. Fill each pocket with half the pesto and half the pine nuts. Place chicken on a small baking dish, which has been coated with vegetable oil spray. With a table knife, spread ½ teaspoon additional pesto sauce on top of each breast, followed by the Parmesan, patting firmly to secure. Gently drizzle ½ teaspoon olive oil over each breast, and bake for approximately 17-20 minutes.

Nightshade free
Gluten free

LEMON CHICKEN ALMONDINE

This simple chicken dish is one of my original 1970s recipes, served at numerous dinner parties through the years. Steamed fresh asparagus is suggested as a side dish. Preheat oven 400 degrees. Serves 8.

8 boneless/skinless chicken breasts
½ cup white wine
2 lemons
1 cup almond slivers, toasted
8 pats butter
½ teaspoon garlic flakes
White pepper and Kosher salt, to taste
1 teaspoon tarragon

In a large shallow baking dish, arrange chicken breasts, in single layer. Pour white wine over chicken, followed by juice of lemons. Zest 1 tablespoon of lemon rind, sprinkle over chicken. Season with garlic flakes, white pepper, salt, and tarragon. Add butter to each breasts, with portion of almonds. Roast uncovered in oven, for approximately 25 minutes, or until chicken is done. Place chicken breasts on large platter, and serve with small bowl of roasting pan juices.

Nightshade free
Gluten free

COG AU VIN

This version of Cog au Vin is a compilation of several recipes. I've added additional vegetables to enhance the stew, altered the traditional bouquet garni, and simplified the process. Preheat oven 350 degrees. Serves 4.

3 tablespoons onion or shallot, minced
3 tablespoons olive oil
10 chicken legs and thighs (with skin and bone)
Kosher salt and black pepper
1 large bay leaf

2 garlic cloves, minced
½ cup fresh parsley, minced
½ teaspoon dried thyme
2 large parsnips, peeled and cut in 1" slices
2 cups small carrots
5 small white onions, whole and peeled
2 ribs celery, sliced
5 mushrooms, sliced
1/3 cup Madeira sherry (and/or 3 tablespoon cognac)
1 cup white wine
1 cup red wine
½ cup water, or as needed

In a large Dutch oven with lid, saute onion in olive oil. Rinse and dry chicken pieces, season with salt and pepper. Add chicken to Dutch oven, turning to brown sides. Add 1-2 tablespoons additional olive oil, if needed. Then add: bay leaf, garlic, parsley, thyme, parsnips, carrots, onions, celery, mushrooms, Madeira sherry, and wines. Add water, if needed. Ingredients should be slightly covered in liquid. Toss gently to distribute seasonings and herbs. Cover and bake 2 -2 ½ hours. Adjust seasons and serve in large, shallow bowls. This dish can be prepared early in the day, or day before.

Nightshade free
Gluten free
Lactose free

EASY CHICKEN VEGETABLE STIR-FRY WITH MADEIRA

Serves 3-4

2 boneless/skinless chicken breasts, cut in thin slices
1/3 cup olive oil
1 tablespoon oregano

½ cup Madeira sherry
¼ cup tamari
Salt and pepper, to taste
1 large carrot, peeled and thinly sliced
2 ribs celery, sliced
1 shallot, minced
2 cups frozen corn, microwave and drained
2 cups frozen green peas, microwave and drained
1 can white kidney beans, rinsed and drained
3 cups cooked brown rice

Place chicken pieces in a bowl with olive oil, oregano, Madeira, tamari, salt and pepper, to taste. Toss well, and refrigerate for 30-45 minutes. Set mixture out 15 minutes before cooking. Place chicken mixture in a large, heated skillet, with lid. Add carrot, celery, shallot, corn, green peas, and white kidney beans. Stir fry until chicken is done, approximately 8-9 minutes. Reduce heat, cover and simmer 2 minutes, to meld flavors. Place over a serving of brown rice.

Nightshade free
Gluten free
Lactose free

CHICKEN WITH ARTICHOKES AND COUSCOUS

Serves 8

4 tablespoons lemon juice
1 teaspoon salt
½ teaspoon pepper
8 boneless/skinless chicken breasts
½ cup olive oil, more as needed
½ cup parsley, minced
2 ½ -3 cups chicken stock

1 teaspoon lemon rind, grated
1 teaspoon cumin
1 cinnamon stick
¼ teaspoon saffron (soaked for 10 min. in ¼ c. water)
1-2 tablespoons fresh ginger, minced
48 green olives, either stuffed with feta or garlic
24 oil packed artichokes hearts, drained well
Couscous, as directed for 8 servings ½ cup each

Mix first 3 ingredients, rub over chicken. In a large skillet or pot, with lid, saute chicken in olive oil, until golden. Remove chicken, and any excess olive oil. Add to skillet: parsley, chicken stock, lemon rind, cumin, cinnamon stick, saffron, and ginger. Mix well, and bring to boil. Add chicken to skillet/pot. Ladle sauce over chicken, cover, simmer for 25 minutes. Add olives and artichokes, mix gently with chicken and sauce. Prepare couscous, according to package directions. In large soup bowls, place ½ cup of couscous in each, followed by a serving of chicken with ample sauce, olives and artichokes. Serve immediately.

Nightshade free
Lactose free

ASIAN CHICKEN STIR-FRY

Serves 4

16 oz. angel hair pasta, cooked (or gluten free pasta)
3-4 tablespoons toasted sesame oil
(plus 1/3 cup toasted sesame oil, for finish)
8-10 mushrooms, sliced (or 2 + cups)
1 cup onion, chopped
5 garlic cloves, minced
½ cup carrot, thinly sliced
1 ½ cups celery, sliced

2 tablespoons fresh ginger. minced
Salt, black and white peppers, to taste
2 cups frozen green peas, cooked and drained
2 cups cooked chicken, diced
Tamari, to taste
1 ½ cups peanuts, dry roasted

Prepare pasta, according to package directions. Place sesame oil in large skillet, add mushrooms, onion, garlic, carrot, celery, and ginger. Saute until vegetables are tender crisp. Add salt and peppers, to taste. Mix well, combine with peas, chicken, and desired amount of pasta. Toss with tamari (to taste), 1/3 cup sesame oil, and peanuts, to finish. Adjust seasonings.

Nightshade free
Gluten free
Lactose free

GINGER CHICKEN

Serves 2.

8-10 chicken tenders
(or 2 boneless/skinless chicken breasts, cut in strips)
¼ cup tamari
3 tablespoons preserved lemon, minced
2 teaspoons ground ginger
Kosher salt and black pepper, to taste
Olive oil

Place chicken tenders in a shallow bowl, with tamari, lemon, ginger, and seasonings. Toss to coat, refrigerate until ready to cook. Add 3 tablespoons olive oil, in a skillet. Heat, saute chicken for 3 minutes, on each side, or until done.

Nightshade free
Gluten free
Lactose free

CHICKEN TENDERS ON GRILL WITH PEPPERCORN HORSHRADISH SAUCE

Preheat gas grill to 400 degrees. Serves 4.

2 packages chicken tenders
(or 4 boneless/skinless chicken breasts, cut in strips)
½ cup tamari
2 tablespoons lemon juice
1/3 cup olive oil
Kosher salt and pepper, to taste
2 teaspoon garlic flakes
1 teaspoon onion powder
Sprigs fresh parsley, for garnish

Mix all ingredients, coating chicken pieces well, marinate for 30 minutes. Grill chicken, approximately 3-4 minutes on each side. As chicken is done, remove from grill and stack to one side of large plate or platter, layering to form a *mound.* Place a small bowl of the following sauce, to one side of chicken mound, for presentation. Tuck sprigs of parsley under chicken, for garnish.

PEPPERCORN HORSERADISH SAUCE

3/4 cup mayonnaise
1 tablespoon Dijon mustard
2-4 tablespoons, horseradish, to taste
1 tablespoon black peppercorn, crushed

Peppercorns can be crushed in a mortar and pestle, or in a small food processor. Mix ingredients well, chill for at least 3 hours. (This sauce is also delicious with fish, pork, beef, and as a condiment for sandwiches, burgers, etc.)

Nightshade free
Gluten free
Lactose free

CHICKEN WITH ASPARAGUS STIR-FRY

Serves 4.

2-3 boneless/skinless chicken breasts, cut in thin slices
2 eggs, beaten
1 lb. fresh asparagus
4 tablespoons tamari
1 tablespoon cornstarch (mixed with ¼ c. cold water)
1/2 cup Madeira sherry
2 teaspoon sesame oil
2-3 tablespoons olive oil
1-2 tablespoons garlic cloves, minced
1 tablespoon fresh ginger, minced (Thai ginger recommended)
1/4 cup chicken stock
1/3 cup chopped scallions
½ cup dry roasted cashews
3 cups cooked brown rice
Kosher salt and white pepper, to taste.

Cut chicken in thin slices, and combine with eggs, set aside. Trim asparagus ends, and cut into 1 ½ inch pieces, set aside. Combine tamari, cornstarch, Madeira, and sesame oil in a bowl, set aside. In large skillet or wok, heat 1-2 tablespoon olive oil, saute garlic and ginger for 2 minutes. Add additional oil, as needed, add chicken and stir-fry until done. To chicken, add asparagus and tamari mixture. Stir to combine and to slightly thicken sauce. To finish, add scallions, cashews, and salt and pepper, to taste. Mix well, and serve over brown rice.

Nightshade free
Gluten free
Lactose

CHICKEN SALAD WITH DRIED CHERRIES AND ALMOND SLIVERS

Need something yummy for a summer picnic? Try this chicken salad enhanced with dried cherries and slivered almonds. Golden raisins can be added, or substituted for the cherries, as well. Serve over a bed of fresh greens, tossed with *Champagne Vinaigrette,* found in *Salads for All Seasons.* Serves 6.

2 12.5 oz. canned chicken breast, drained
½ to ¾ cup dried pitted cherries, coarsely chopped (or ½ to ¾ cup golden raisins)
½ cup slivered almonds, toasted
½ cup sweet pickle relish
3 hard boiled eggs, diced
3 ribs celery, chopped
1 cup mayonnaise
Kosher salt and pepper, to taste

Mix all the ingredients well. Plate over salad greens.

Nightshade free
Gluten free
Lactose free

CLASSIC CHICKEN AND DUMPLINGS

My friend, Kathy, from Germantown, Tennessee, makes the most incredible chicken and dumplings. She shares her recipe, but never pass an opportunity to sit at her table when she's serving this classic dish.
Serves 6.

CHICKEN PREPARATION
1 whole hen
½ cup dehydrated onions
2 bay leaves
1-2 tablespoons whole black peppercorns

Kosher salt and pepper
Water to almost cover hen

Salt and pepper hen (cavity and outside), place in a crock pot, or in a large, stock pot, with lid. (If using a stock pot, add more water.) Add onions, bay leaves, peppercorns, and water. Cook for several hours in a crock pot, or simmer on the stove for approximately one hour. When very tender, remove hen from broth. When cooled, bone the meat. Salt and pepper chicken, to taste. Refrigerate chicken and broth separately. Skim fat from broth, when thoroughly chilled.

DUMPLINGS
2 cups flour
1 teaspoon salt
1 ½ teaspoon baking powder
2 tablespoons oil
½ cup 2% lactose free milk (for dough)
1 egg, beaten
½ cup 2% lactose free milk, warmed, with 1 T. flour
1 can *undiluted* cream of chicken soup, optional
Green scallions, sliced (garnish)

Sift flour, blend with salt and baking powder. Whisk oil, ½ cup milk, and egg. Mix dry and liquid ingredients well. Roll out dough (about ¼ inch thick), on a floured cutting board, and cut into strips. Place broth in large pan, bring to a boil. Drop dumplings, one at a time, into bubbling broth and cook 10 minutes uncovered. Maintain gentle boil. Dumplings may be crowded, but gently stir several times. Cover and cook 10 additional minutes. About halfway through the second 10 minutes, add ½ cup warm milk (mixed with 1 T. flour), and the boned chicken meat. Cover, and continue to cook. As an option, add can of *undiluted* cream of chicken soup to broth, for added richness. Serve in soup bowls, with green scallions.

Nightshade free
Lactose free

FRIED CHICKEN LIVERS WITH SHERRY SAUCE

This is another Southern classic dish, served with a luscious Madeira sherry sauce. When making the sauce, be sure to include some of the crusty flour sediment that has fallen to the bottom of pan. This dish is lovely for Sunday brunch, served with champagne and strawberries. Serves 4.

Package of chicken livers, 12-15 pieces
Kosher salt and black pepper, to taste
Flour
Peanut or canola oil

Rinse and dry livers, lay on a clean, flat surface. With a toothpick or other sharp object, prick each liver several times, to help eliminate splatters during frying process. Salt and pepper, to taste, dredge in flour. In a deep skillet, and 1 inch *hot* oil, place livers in a single layer, slightly covered. Do not crowd. Turn livers, to brown and crisp all sides, 3-5 minutes. When done, remove to paper towels. For sauce, follow instructions below:

MADEIRA SHERRY SAUCE
4 tablespoons cooking oil from pan (with crusty sediment)
3-4 tablespoons flour
2 % lactose free milk (1-2 cups, as needed)
Kosher salt and black pepper, to taste
¼-½ cup Madeira sherry

Pour off excess oil, reserve 4 tablespoons and crusty sediment. Reheat to a gentle sizzle. Add flour to oil, stir to cook and form paste. Slowly add and whisk milk, until very smooth. For desired consistency, add as much milk as needed. Add Madeira, salt and pepper, blending well. Bring to a gentle boil, and serve with chicken livers.

Nightshade free
Lactose free

BEEF AND PORK TO FEED BODY AND SOUL

BEEF AND PORK TO FEED BODY AND SOUL

For many of us, there is nothing that satisfies like beef or pork. Whether it's a simple steak on the grill, seasoned well and cooked to perfection, or a celebratory meal with family or friends, beef and pork are hard to beat. For those times, here are a few hearty recipes to sample.

COCONUT MEATBALLS WITH RASPBERRIES IN THE SNOW

The distinct flavors of this spicy dish, and the final garnish, makes this recipe a winner. Curry powders, without nightshades, are available at specialty spice shops, and usually come in several varieties. Serves 4.

1 lb. ground sirloin
Curry powder, without nightshades
1 egg, beaten
2-3 garlic cloves, minced
1 teaspoon salt
1 teaspoon white pepper
½ teaspoon black pepper
½ cup fresh parsley, chopped
½ cup sweetened coconut, grated
3 tablespoons olive oil
2 cups light sweetened coconut milk
(add 1 teaspoon curry powder)
4 servings fresh broccoli
(lightly steamed with salt, pepper, 1 t. butter, 3 T. water)

Handful cilantro, chopped
Garnish: *Raspberries in the Snow* (see below)

Mix sirloin with:1 tablespoon curry powder, egg, garlic, salt, peppers, parsley, and coconut. Roll into small meatballs. Slowly heat oil in skillet to medium-high. Meanwhile, place coconut milk and curry in small pan to slightly thicken, set aside. Steam broccoli, set aside. When oil is hot, fry meatballs in skillet, until crisp. Drain on paper towel. On 4 plates, add a serving of broccoli, followed by a serving of meatballs, and 2-3 tablespoons of coconut milk mixture. Top with 2 tablespoons cilantro. For *Raspberries in the Snow,* place 2 tablespoons of grated coconut in center of each serving to form a small *nest*, followed by 3-5 fresh raspberries. Serve immediately.

Nightshade free
Gluten free
Lactose free (omit butter in broccoli)

MEATLOAF WITH VEGETABLES

Most of us grew up eating meatloaf at least once a month. It's still a family favorite, but this recipe is laced with vegetables. The vegetables are chopped (not minced) and added raw to the meatloaf, for texture and more vegetable flavor. For smoother texture, lightly saute vegetables before adding to meatloaf. *Corn Rice Cheese Bake,* in chapter *Savory Pastas and Grains,* is recommended as a side dish. Place rack in middle of oven and preheat to 375 degrees. Serves 6-8.

2 medium onions, chopped
1-2 tablespoon garlic, minced
2-3 medium celery ribs, chopped
1 large carrot, chopped
4 scallions, sliced
2 teaspoon salt

2 teaspoon coarse black pepper
½ teaspoon white pepper
3 tablespoons Worcestershire sauce (without chili extract)
2 tablespoons balsamic vinegar
2 ½ pounds ground beef (freshly ground and lean)
1 cup Italian bread crumbs
2 large eggs, lightly beaten
1/3 cup fresh parsley, minced

Place rack in middle of preheated oven. Mix all ingredients gently, using a tossing motion with your hands, so not to over mix or pack down. Carefully form mixture into a 10x5 inch loaf, then place in 13x9 inch baking pan. Bake until center temperature reaches 155 degrees, with outer edges browned or approximately 1 ½ hours. Let meatloaf stand, covered loosely with foil for 10 minutes before serving.

Nightshade free
Lactose free

SPINACH STUFFED BEEF TENDERLOIN ROAST

Looking for something special for a holiday party? Try this recipe for beef tenderloin roast. The stuffing adds the perfect touch, and it's a grand centerpiece on any buffet. When ready to roast, preheat oven to 425 degrees. Serves 12.

1 ½ cups favorite vinaigrette
3 ½ lb. beef tenderloin roast
2 tablespoons olive oil
½ lb. fresh mushrooms, coarsely chopped
4 green onions, sliced
2-3 garlic cloves, minced
20 oz. fresh spinach
1/3 cup pine nuts
1 teaspoon Kosher salt

¼ teaspoon onion powder
½ teaspoon white pepper
½ black pepper
Extra black pepper, for exterior of roast

Rinse and dry the beef tenderloin roast, trim excess fat, place in a container, with lid. Pour vinaigrette over roast, covering all sides, close container, and refrigerate overnight. Remove meat from refrigerator one hour before cooking, do not blot marinade. Preheat oven before cooking spinach mixture. In a medium skillet, add olive oil, mushrooms, onions, garlic, spinach, pint nuts, salt, onion powder, and both peppers. Saute until mushrooms are cooked and spinach is wilted. Use paper towels to absorb excess moisture in skillet. Cut a slit down center of roast to within ¾ inch of bottom. Open meat on a flat working surfaces. Spread spinach filling over one side of meat, fold other side over stuffing. Tie several times with kitchen string to secure. Sprinkle surface of meat with black pepper, place tenderloin on a shallow roasting pan. Cook uncovered, in center of oven, at 425 degrees for 40-55 minutes, or until meat thermometer reaches desired doneness (for medium-rare to 145 degrees; medium to 160 degrees; well-done to170 degrees). Let stand for 10 minutes. Remove string before slicing and serving.

Nightshade free
Gluten free
Lactose free

FILET OF BEEF TENDERLOIN

Preheat gas grill to 475-500 degrees. Serves 4.

4 beef tenderloin filets, rinsed and dried
(4-6 oz. each, about 1 ½ + inches thick)
1/3 cup olive oil
Salt and black pepper, to taste
½ + teaspoon garlic flakes

½ + teaspoon onion powder
1-2 tablespoon fresh lemon juice
2 tablespoons tamari (or 2 tablespoons balsamic vinegar)
Black peppercorn, finely crushed (optional)

Place steaks in a shallow dish. Mix remaining ingredients, spread over steaks. Turn meat several times, to heavily coat. Add additional olive oil, if needed. Refrigerate for 1-3 hours, set out 1 hour prior to cooking. Preheat grill. High heat is a necessary component for a great steak, and cooking time varies according to size and thickness. A rule of thumb for rare is 2 minutes (or less) on each side.

Nightshade free
Gluten free
Lactose free

STUFFED ZUCCHINI AND SIRLOIN

Preheat oven to 375 degrees. Serves 2.

2 large zucchini, cut in half with both ends attached
4 tablespoons ground sirloin
1 tablespoon olive oil
2 tablespoons onion, minced
2 tablespoons celery, minced
Salt, black and white peppers, to taste
½ teaspoon garlic flakes
½ cup mozzarella cheese, grated

Scoop flesh from zucchini carefully, chop. Place zucchini flesh, ground sirloin, olive oil, onion, celery, and seasonings, in a small skillet. Sauté slightly, but do not brown meat. Stuff zucchini halves with mixture, and place in a shallow dish. Top with cheese, and bake for approximately 35-45 minutes, or until zucchini is tender, but not limp.

Nightshade free
Gluten free

BOEUF BOURGUIGNON

This lovely French stew is rich in flavor and is enhanced by red wine and vegetables. If desired, additional black pepper adds a spicy touch.
Serves 4-6.

3 lbs. stew meat, rinsed and dried
Kosher salt and pepper, to taste
2 cups flour
Vegetable oil
½ cup dry vermouth
4 large parsnips, peeled and sliced in 1 ½ pieces (parsnips adds a touch of sweetness to stew)
3-4 cups small carrots
10-12 large mushrooms, quartered
2 ribs celery, sliced in ¾ inch pieces
4-5 garlic cloves, minced
2 white onions, sliced in wedges
1 bay leaf
2 teaspoon dried thyme
1/8 teaspoon ground cloves
3 tablespoons dried parsley
1 bottle dry red wine
3-4 cups beef stock, or as needed

Season dried stew meat with ample salt and pepper, dredge in bowl of flour. In a large pot, add 3-4 tablespoons of vegetable oil, heat, add meat in batches to thoroughly brown. Add additional oil, if needed. Do not crowd meat while browning, or allow flour residue to burn. When nicely browned, place meat in a bowl. Pour vermouth in stew pot to deglaze pan, scraping crusty bits from sides. Pour pan contents over meat. In same pan, add 3-4 tablespoons additional oil, parsnips, carrots, mushrooms, celery, garlic, and onions. Over medium heat, cook vegetables for 10 minutes, or until onion begins to caramelize. Add bay leaf, thyme, cloves, and parsley. Add red wine and

2 cups of beef stock, to cover contents of pot. Bring to boil, reduce heat to simmer. Cover slightly, and simmer for 3 ½ - 4 hours, or until stew meat is very tender. Add additional beef stock, as necessary. Adjust seasonings, cool. Stew can be served same day, but flavor greatly improves if refrigerated overnight. When ready to serve, heat thoroughly.

Nightshade free
Lactose free

GOLABKI (POLISH STUFFED CABBAGE ROLLS) WITH MUSHROOM AND ONION SAUCE

This delicious classic recipe is shared by my friend Marysia. It's a sumptuous dish. Serves 6-8.

1 large head cabbage
2 cups cooked rice
1 lb. lean ground beef
2 teaspoon salt
2 cloves garlic, minced
3 tablespoon onion, minced
¾ teaspoon white pepper
½ teaspoon black pepper
1 egg, beaten
Quart chicken stock

Cut core from cabbage, place in a large pot of water. Cover and bring to boil. Reduce heat to medium high, cook for 10 minutes. Remove cabbage carefully from water, let stand for 1 hour, or run under cold water to cool. Carefully remove leaves of cabbage (which usually release from the head easily), set aside. If necessary, cut veins from leaves, for more flexibility. (Save any torn leaves, for placement in bottom of cooking pot.) For meat stuffing, mix remaining ingredients, except chicken stock. Take each leaf in hand, add an oval shaped ball of meat mixture to center. Fold in sides, roll leaf to secure. Place in bottom of a large deep pan, with lid. Repeat process until all leaves and meat mixture are used. Cabbage rolls need to be tightly arranged in pan. If there are extra whole leaves, place on top of cabbage rolls, salt and pepper lightly. Add chicken stock, to almost cover rolls. Bring to boil, then reduce to simmer. Cover and cook for 1 ½ - 2 hours. Add more stock or water, as needed. (For presentation, arrange any extra cooked leaves on platter, then place cabbage rolls on top.)

MUSHROOM SAUCE

¼ -1/3 cup butter
10-15 mushrooms, sliced
1 medium onion, finely diced
3 tablespoons flour
1-2 cups 2 % lactose free milk
Chicken stock or water, as needed
Kosher salt and pepper, to taste

In large skillet, melt butter, add mushrooms and onion. Saute until tender. While stirring, add flour and cook until a paste forms. Slowly add milk, and continue, mixing well. To thin sauce, add additional milk, chicken stock, or water. Season well, with salt and pepper. When ready to serve, place cabbage rolls on serving plate, add a tablespoon of sauce over each roll. Serve immediately. Pass additional sauce at the table.

Nightshade Free

PORK TENDERLOIN WITH FOUR SAUCES

High cooking temperatures create a lovely outer crust for this pork tenderloin recipe, while maintaining the juices. There are many sauces that enhance pork tenderloin, but four favorites are included below. Pork tenderloin is nightshade, gluten and lactose free. The sauces are as indicated. Serves 8-10.

PORK TENDERLOIN PREPARATION

Rinse and dry pork, then place in a shallow dish. Follow with an ample amount of *Caroline's Dry Spicy Rub,* listed in *Beverages, Sauces, and Other Fun Stuff.* Press rub into flesh of pork, as desired. The more rub used, the spicier the pork. Refrigerate for 5-6 hours. Set out 30 minutes prior to cooking.

Preheat gas grill to 400-450 degrees, or oven to 450 degrees. Cook to desired doneness, 20-25 minutes, depending on size of tenderloin. Pork should be brown and crisp on the outside, and slightly pink and juicy inside. Let stand 10-15 minutes, loosely tented with foil, before slicing.

FOUR SAUCES FOR PORK TENDERLOIN

1. Cherry Sauce Makes about 1 cup.
Heat 1-2 tablespoons vegetable oil in a small skillet. Add and saute:
1 shallot, minced; and 1 garlic clove, minced. Add ½ cup sweet vermouth. Bring to boil. Add 1 can pitted cherries, drained, or 1 ½ cups frozen pitted cherries, thawed. Add 1/4 cup agave or sugar (to taste), then simmer until sauce thickens. Season with pinch of salt and black pepper.
Nightshade, gluten, and lactose free

2. Dried Apricot Sauce Makes about 1 cup.
Place 6 ounces of dried apricots cut in pieces (or pears, apples, or other dried fruit), in a small sauce pan, with ¾ cup port and ½ cup orange juice. Bring to boil, then reduce heat to simmer for 8-10 minutes, until fruit is poached and sauce thickens. For a sweeter sauce, add agave or sugar, to taste.
Nightshade, gluten, and lactose free

3. Prune and Madeira Sauce Makes about 1 ½ cups.
Cut 1 cup dried prunes, in quarters. Place prunes, 2 tablespoons butter, and ½ teaspoon dried rosemary, in a small sauce pan or skillet, lightly saute. Add

¾ cup Madeira sherry, ½ cup water, and ½ cup orange marmalade. Simmer until slightly thickened.
Nightshade and gluten free

4. Oriental Sauce with Fresh Red Cabbage
Prepare a bed of chopped red cabbage (about 2 cups), spread on serving platter. When pork tenderloin is sliced and ready to serve, arrange in a circle on cabbage. Add a small bowl of your favorite Asian sauce, in center of pork. Specialty oriental sauces are available commercially at many groceries. Serve pork tenderloin with mini-buns or petite rolls, for party sandwiches.
Nightshade and lactose free

HAM AND ASPARAGUS ROLL-UPS

My friend, Carol, serves this delicious and elegant dish at luncheons. However, this entrée would be a luscious addition to any brunch, as well. Preheat oven to 350 degrees. Serves 8.

24 fresh asparagus spears
8 pieces ham, thinly sliced
8 pieces Swiss cheese, thinly sliced
12 oz. light cream cheese, softened
¼ cup milk
½ cup Parmesan cheese
½ teaspoon dried parsley flakes
(or 1 tablespoon fresh parsley, minced)
3 oz. sliced almonds
Salt and pepper, to taste

Wash asparagus and trim tough ends. Pre-cook asparagus 2 minutes in the microwave. Place 1 slice of cheese on each piece of ham. Roll ham and cheese around 3 asparagus spears, place in 8x12 baking dish. Bake for 15 minutes. Combine cream cheese, milk, Parmesan, and parsley, beat well. Add salt and pepper, if desired. Remove roll-ups from oven, add sauce, sprinkle with almonds, and bake an additional 10 minutes.

Nightshade free

Gluten free

BRATWURST WITH CABBAGE AND APPLES

This hearty stew is perfect for casual, winter gatherings, and is a colorful main course. Sweet potatoes and apple provide a touch of sweetness to this savory dish. Serves 6.

6 slices bacon, fried and crumbled
1 onion, chopped
1-2 cloves garlic, minced
4 cups green cabbage, coarsely sliced
2 medium sweet potatoes, peeled and diced
1 cup water
¾ cup white wine, or apple juice
1 tablespoon brown sugar
1 teaspoon chicken bouillon
1 teaspoon caraway seed
1 bay leaf
1 pound bratwurst, cut in 1 ½ in pieces
1 large apple, cored and sliced

Fry bacon, crumble, set aside. In a large pot, cook onion and garlic, in 2 tablespoons drippings from frying bacon. Add cabbage, sweet potatoes, water, white wine or apple juice, brown sugar, bouillon, caraway seed, and bay leaf. Mix well, bring to boil. Add bratwurst pieces to the pot, cover, and simmer for 1-1 ¼ hours. Add additional water, as needed. To finish, add apple, and cook last 10 minutes, or until tender. Remove bay leaf, add crumbled bacon, and serve.

Nightshade free

Gluten free

Lactose free

LOVELY VEGETABLES AND VEGETARIAN ENTREES

LOVELY VEGETABLES AND VEGETARIAN ENTREES

When I think of my favorite vegetables, I no longer include tomatoes, peppers of all types and colors, white potatoes, or eggplant. These nightshade vegetables are now replaced with delicious other choices, that I find just as satisfying as the nightshades from my past. It was a challenge at first, to be honest, but I no longer miss them. Having relief from arthritis pain and inflammation in my hands, is worth much more than a few bites of foods that cause me severe discomfort for hours, sometimes days.

Sweet potatoes are featured in many of the recipes that follow, either as replacements for white potatoes, or as main ingredients. Sweet potatoes are more nutritious than white potatoes, and complement many other vegetables in casseroles, etc. Although, a distant relative of the nightshades, sweet potatoes are not a member of the *Solanaceae* family, and therefore, can be safely eaten and enjoyed by anyone sensitive to nightshades.

In this chapter, you will find not only interesting vegetable dishes, but also vegetarian entrees that are nightshade free, and often gluten and lactose free.

ROSEMARY SWEET POTATO MASH

Serves 6-8.

3-4 medium sweet potatoes, peeled and cut in ½ in. slices
Water to cover potatoes, plus 1 inch
½ teaspoon salt
1 teaspoon black pepper

3 teaspoons dried rosemary, crushed
1-2 teaspoon cumin
½ teaspoon garlic flakes
¼ cup half and half
3 tablespoons softened light cream cheese
½ cup Parmesan cheese

Place sweet potatoes, water, salt, and black pepper in a large pot, bring to boil. Reduce heat, cover slightly, and cook until tender, approximately 25 minutes. Drain well. Mash potatoes with remaining ingredients. Add additional salt and black pepper, to taste.

Nightshade free
Gluten free

GARLIC SWEET POTATOES "FRIES"

Preheat oven to 400 degrees. Serves 4-6.

Vegetable oil spray
3 medium sweet potatoes, peeled
Salt and black pepper, to taste
Garlic flakes
1 teaspoon dried oregano
1/2 cup olive oil
Ranch dressing

Cover large cookie sheet with foil, coat with vegetable oil spray. Slice sweet potatoes in a thick "French fry cut." Place in a large bowl, toss with remaining ingredients, and spread on cookie sheet. Bake for approximately 35-40 minutes, or until sweet potatoes are tender, brown, and crisp. Serve immediately with ranch dressing.

Nightshade free
Gluten free
Lactose free

CORN PUDDING

This is my friend Susan's historic corn pudding recipe that was enjoyed at Kentucky family holidays for several generations. It is amazing and is now featured at our holiday table as well. The recipe originally came from: Woodford Chapter DAR, Limestone Chapter, *Kentucky Heritage Cookbook,* Maysville, Kentucky. In 1810, this recipe was featured at Kentucky's revered Paxton Inn. Preheat oven to 350-375 degrees. 5-6 servings.

3 eggs
2 cups whole milk and half and half, equal parts mix
2 ½ cups frozen corn, thaw (or fresh, removed from cob)
3 tablespoons sugar, or less
2 tablespoons butter, melted
Salt, to taste
1 tablespoon flour

Whisk eggs. In a food processor, add ½ cup corn, with a little milk, to slightly smooth. Scrape into a small sauce pan to warm. Add this mixture and remaining corn, to the eggs. Follow with sugar, butter, salt, and flour, blending well between each addition. Butter large casserole dish, fill with corn mixture. Bake for 45 minutes to 1 hour. Stir casserole a couple times during baking process. Corn pudding will be golden brown when done. This recipe doubles well.

Nightshade free
Gluten free

VEGGIE RELISH

This simple dish is a perfect side dish for cookouts, picnics, pot lucks, and other casual gatherings. It's also great for your next football party, served with lime corn chips. Serves 8 as side dish, or 10-12 as appetizer.

1 can hominy, rinsed and drained
1 can corn, drained

1 can black beans, rinsed and drained
1 large carrot, peeled and thinly sliced
2 ribs celery, chopped
½ cup onion, minced
2 green onions, sliced
4 radishes, sliced
Salt, black and white peppers, to taste
1 teaspoon garlic flakes
1 teaspoon cumin
White pepper, to taste
¾ cup your favorite vinaigrette

Mix all ingredients in a large bowl, and adjust seasonings, to taste. Serve at room temperature.

Nightshade free
Gluten free
Lactose free

ROASTED CABBAGE

Simple recipe, but this is the way to enjoy cabbage. Once tasted, you'll always want it roasted. Preheat oven to 375-400 degrees. Serves 8.

Vegetable oil spray
1 large head green cabbage
1 large onion, sliced
Kosher salt and pepper, to taste
Olive oil, or flavor enhanced olive oil
Dried Italian herb mix, or oregano

Line a large cookie sheet with foil, lightly coated with vegetable oil spray. Slice and arrange cabbage and onion, on foil. Salt and pepper, to taste. Drizzle olive oil and sprinkle herbs, over the cabbage. Roast in oven, until slightly crisp and tender, approximately 45-50 minutes. Note: Leftover Roasted

Cabbage can easily become a delightful pureed soup. Please see: *Succulent Soups and Stews* for *Puree of Roasted Cabbage and Onion Soup.*
Nightshade free
Gluten free
Lactose free

ROASTED VEGETABLE MIX

This recipe is similar to the Roasted Cabbage recipe above, but with a hearty mix of additional vegetables. Again, roasting is the key component.
Preheat oven to 400 degrees. Serves 8-10.

Vegetable oil spray
3 beets, peeled and diced
4 large carrots, peeled and cut in 1 inch pieces
1 large onion, cut in wedges
10 whole garlic cloves
3 celery ribs, cut in 1 inch pieces
1-2 sweet potatoes, peeled and diced
Olive oil
2 tablespoons dried Italian herb mix
Salt and black pepper, to taste

Line a large cookie sheet with foil, and lightly coat with vegetable oil spray. Combine all vegetables in a large bowl, toss with ample olive oil, salt, pepper, and herbs. Roast on cookie sheet, for approximately 45 minutes to 1 hour. When sweet potatoes and beets are tender and slightly browned, serve warm or room temperature.
Nightshade free
Gluten free
Lactose free

BRUSSELS SPROUTS WITH WALNUTS, APPLES, AND RAISINS

This luscious recipe comes from my Oklahoma City friend, Pat, who serves this special Provencal dish with turkey during the holidays, or any other festive occasion. Serves 2.

10 oz. fresh Brussels sprouts
1 teaspoon sea salt
1 tablespoon olive oil
½ large onion, thinly sliced
1 garlic clove, thinly sliced
1 large Rome apple, cut in 1 inch pieces
Pinch sugar
½ teaspoon grated lemon zest
¼ cup walnuts
¼ cup golden raisins
Pinch freshly ground nutmeg
Freshly ground black pepper and salt, to taste
½ teaspoon unsalted butter

Bring Brussels sprouts to boil in salted water. Cook about 10 minutes. Drain, rinse in cold water, cut in half lengthwise, set aside. In a medium skillet, add olive oil, onion, garlic, apple, sugar, lemon zest, walnuts, raisins, nutmeg, pepper, and salt. Saute for 5 minutes. Add cooked Brussels sprouts to skillet, and cook 5 additional minutes. Toss with butter, and serve hot.

Nightshade free
Gluten free
Lactose free (omit butter)

SOUTHERN (SWEET) POTATO SALAD

Potato salad has been a spring and summer standard in our family for decades. However, this potato salad is made with sweet potatoes, the *no nightshade potato,* and would be a winner with ham, deviled eggs, and corn pudding on Easter Sunday. The recipe is found in *Salads for All Seasons.*

NAPA CABBAGE AND ONION STIR- FRY

Serves 2-3.

½ head Napa cabbage, sliced
1 onion, sliced
4 mushrooms, sliced
Olive oil
Kosher salt and pepper, to taste
1 teaspoon oregano

Place all ingredients in a medium skillet. Stir fry for a few minutes, or until vegetables wilt, slightly. Serve as a side dish or as a garnish for fish, chicken, or pork.

Nightshade free
Gluten free
Lactose free

TURNIP AND SWEET POTATO MASH WITH GOAT CHEESE

Serves 4-5.

3 sweet potatoes, peeled and sliced
1 turnip, peeled and sliced
Water
1 tablespoon oregano
4 rounded tablespoons goat cheese, softened
Kosher salt and pepper, to taste

Cover sweet potatoes and turnip with water, and a pinch of salt and pepper. Bring to boil, reduce heat, cover, and simmer for 25 minutes, or until tender.

Drain well. Add oregano, goat cheese, salt and pepper, mash well. Serve as a side dish with meat, chicken, or pork.
Nightshade free
Gluten free

ARTICHOKE STEAMED WITH VINAIGRETTE

A recipe for fresh, steamed artichoke is found in *Appetizers for Festive Starts.* If serving as a first course at a dinner party, provide one whole artichoke for each guest.

PUREE OF PARSNIPS WITH SCOTCH WHISKEY

Serves 6-8.

2 lbs. parsnips, peeled and thinly sliced
1 onion, coarsely chopped
4 tablespoons butter, softened
1-2 cups chicken stock
water
1 oz. scotch whiskey
1 teaspoon nutmeg
Kosher salt

In a medium pot, place parsnips over onions, add 2 tablespoons butter, chicken stock, and water to cover (2 inches above vegetables). Simmer until very soft, approximately 30-45 minutes. Add water, if necessary. When done, the liquid should be mostly evaporated. Place parsnip mix in food processor (or use a stick blender in the same pot), with some of the broth. Add remainder of butter, scotch, nutmeg, and salt, to taste. Puree until smooth. Serve immediately.
Nightshade free
Gluten free

SCALLOPED TURNIPS

Preheat oven to 375 degrees. Serves 4-6.

In this recipe, the brilliant white color of the turnips, contrasted by the dark flakes of basil, creates an elegant and fragrant side dish. Turnip is a vegetable that is often overlooked, but is versatile, and a delicious addition to the table.

3 large turnips, peeled and sliced
½ teaspoon salt
½ teaspoon white pepper
1 teaspoon ground dry mustard
2 teaspoons dried basil
1 ½ cups (total) half and half / 1 % milk mix
3 tablespoons butter

Combine salt, pepper, dry mustard, and basil, with the milk mixture. Layer half the turnips in a covered casserole. Pour half the liquid over the turnips, and repeat layer. Add dollops of the butter on top. Cover and bake 45-50 minutes, until tender.

Nightshade free
Gluten free

CASHEW, KALE, AND VEGGIE STIR- FRY

Serves 4 as main course.

1 cup brown rice, cooked and set aside
3 tablespoons olive oil
3 garlic cloves, minced
½ cup onion
1 tablespoon (each) water and tamari
1 teaspoon white pepper
½ teaspoon salt
1 ½ cups carrots, chopped
2 cups mushrooms, sliced

1 bunch Kale, stems removed and coarsely chopped
1 quarter preserved lemon, minced
½ head Napa cabbage
½ cup cashews (garnish)
½ cup cilantro, chopped (garnish)

In an oversized skillet, add olive oil, sauté garlic and onion, until translucent. Add water, tamari, pepper, salt, carrots, mushrooms, kale, preserved lemon, and Napa cabbage. Stir-fry until ingredients are tender crisp. Add additional tamari, if moisture is needed. Toss with 1-2 cups cooked rice, for desired volume. Place in a large bowl, garnish with the cilantro and cashews. Serve immediately.

Nightshade free
Gluten free
Lactose free

GREEN VEGETABLE STIR- FRY WITH QUINOA

Serves 8 as main course.

4 tablespoons olive oil
4-5 garlic cloves, minced
½ large onion, chopped
3 tablespoons fresh ginger, minced (Thai Ginger, if available)
6-8 cups fresh spinach, packed down
3 cups green cabbage, sliced, then cut in half
2 cups asparagus, cut in 2 inch pieces
½ cup celery, sliced
1 can black beans, rinsed and drained
I can garbanzo beans, rinsed and drained
3 tablespoon tamari
Salt, white and black peppers, to taste
½ cup cashews

1 cup quinoa, cook and set aside
Fresh parsley or cilantro, for garnish

In a large skillet with lid, sauté garlic, onion, and ginger, in olive oil. Add the remaining ingredients, except quinoa and cashews. Stir-fry, lifting the vegetables and ingredients to mix well and to distribute heat. Add additional tamari and olive oil, if needed. When done, toss contents of skillet with cashews and 1-2 cups of cooked quinoa, as desired. Serve immediately. Garnish with fresh parsley or cilantro. Offer additional tamari at table.

Nightshade free
Gluten free
Lactose free

NEW YEAR'S DAY BLACK-EYED PEAS

This casserole was inspired by *Hopping John,* that was popular in the 1980s, on New Year's Day. This is a vegetarian adaptation without nightshades, gluten or lactose, which can be served as a main course or side dish. It brings good luck for the New Year, either way. Serves 10-12.

1 pound dried black-eyed peas, rinsed well and picked over (cook according to directions on package)
½ cup leek, sliced thinly
1 cup brown rice, cooked and set aside
Black and white peppers, abundant, or to taste
Salt, to taste
1 tablespoon Italian herb mix
1 tablespoon garlic flakes
2 teaspoon thyme
2 teaspoons sage
1/3 cup olive oil, or flavor enhanced olive oil (plus extra for finish)
½ cup parsley, minced

¾ cup carrot, minced
2 ribs celery, minced

While peas are cooking, add the leek. When peas and leek are tender (approximately 45-55 minutes), drain and add remaining ingredients quickly, to retain heat. Mix well, but do not mash. Cover pot for 10 minutes to partially steam vegetables and blend seasoning flavors. Vegetables will be tender crisp. Add cooked rice (in preferred amount), tossing gently. Adjust seasonings, including herbs. Loosely place mixture, in a large casserole dish, lightly drizzle with additional olive oil.

Nightshade free
Gluten free
Lactose free

VEGETABLE RHAPSODY

Rhapsody casseroles were original vegetarian creations that our family enjoyed in the late 1980s. These casseroles were packed with nightshades, but today's version is nightshade free and gluten free. This is a healthy main course or side dish, full of nutritional, colorful vegetables, and surprising tastes. Preheat oven 400 degrees. Serves 4-6.

1 large sweet potato, peeled and thinly sliced
½ onion, chopped
2 turnips, peeled and thinly sliced
2 large carrots, peeled and thinly sliced
1-2 zucchini, sliced ½ inch thick
3 cups cabbage, thinly sliced
1/2 cup tamari
1 teaspoon garlic flakes
1-2 tablespoon Italian herb mix
Kosher salt and black pepper, to taste
1 cup Parmesan, grated

Coat a large casserole with vegetable oil spray. Layer half of the vegetables, add half the tamari, seasonings, and Parmesan. Repeat second layer, slightly press down vegetables. Cover and bake approximately 50 minutes, or until vegetables are tender throughout casserole.

Nightshade free

Gluten free

CREAMED SPINACH AND MUSHROOM CASSEROLE

My friend, Cathy, shared her recipe for creamed spinach, which I've incorporated in the recipe below. This particular style of spinach can also be served as a side dish, or topping for polenta or pasta. Preheat broiler to high. Serves 4.

12-14 white mushrooms, sliced
2 tablespoons olive oil
Salt and pepper, to taste
Vegetable oil spray
2 tablespoons butter
6-8 cups fresh spinach, packed down
½ teaspoon nutmeg
5 eggs, beaten
1 cup Parmesan cheese, grated

In large skillet, saute mushrooms, slightly seasoned with salt and pepper, in 2 tablespoons olive oil. Cook until browned slightly, and water evaporates. Drain if necessary. Place mushrooms in a large pie plate, coated with vegetable oil spray. Keep warm. In same skillet, add 2 tablespoons butter, spinach, and nutmeg, lightly season with salt and pepper, over medium high heat. Toss ingredients with tongs to completely wilt spinach. Add eggs and ¾ cup Parmesan to spinach, mixing well, and to set eggs. Place mixture over mushrooms in pie plate. Add additional Parmesan on top, place under broiler, until cheese browns. Divide into four servings.

Nightshade free
Gluten free

RED BEANS AND RICE

Hungry for something hot and spicy, but without nightshade pain and inflammation? Try this recipe for *Red Beans and Rice*. This version is abundantly seasoned with white and black peppers, which are not nightshades. If you want it hotter, just increase the white pepper. File (pronounced *fee-lay)* is an American Indian herb which has been adopted by Cajun chefs. File, not only thickens, but adds a subtle, distinctive flavor to soups, beans, gumbos, etc. Serves 6.

1 cup Calrose rice, cooked
16 oz. red beans, soaked 6 hours in water
1 qt. chicken stock
5 garlic cloves, minced
1 large onion, chopped
1 cup celery, thinly sliced
1 cup carrot, chopped
2 cups okra (fresh or frozen)
1 teaspoon white pepper, or more
1 teaspoon black pepper, or more
Salt, to taste
1-2 teaspoon file

Drain beans after soaking, cover with fresh water, 2 inches above beans. Add chicken stock, garlic, onion, celery, carrot, okra, peppers, and salt. Bring to boil, reduce heat to high simmer. Cover, and cook until beans are tender, approximately 1 ½ hours. Do not over cook beans. Add 1 teaspoon file at a time, to determine desired thickening. Adjust seasonings and add cooked rice, as preferred.

Nightshade free

Gluten free
Lactose free

SWEET POTATOES AND SPINACH IN SPICED ORANGE SAUCE

Having been an avid fan of Mollie Katzen's cookbooks over the years, I was delighted when my friend, Patrice, offered this special recipe from Mollie's, *Vegetable Haven.* This is a lovely nightshade, gluten, and lactose free dish. Serves 6-8.

2-3 tablespoons vegetable oil
3 cups onion, chopped (2 medium)
3 tablespoons Persian allspice
(see below or use regular allspice)
2 ½ teaspoons garlic, minced
8 cups cubed sweet potatoes or yams (about 3 lbs.)
3 cups orange juice
1 teaspoon salt
1 ½ cups prunes, pitted and sliced
1-2 lbs. fresh spinach, as desired
(or 2 boxes 10 oz. frozen spinach)

In a large pot or Dutch oven, heat oil, add onion and Persian allspice. Saute about 5 minutes over medium heat. Stir in garlic, sweet potatoes or yams, orange juice, and salt. Mix well. Cover and cook over medium heat until potatoes are tender, about 25-30 minutes. Add prunes and spinach, stirring well. Cover and cook over low heat for 10 minutes.

PERSIAN ALLSPICE
Mix the following ingredients well.
1 teaspoon salt
1 tablespoon coriander
1 teaspoon cardamom

1 tablespoon cumin
2 teaspoons cinnamon
2 teaspoons turmeric
2 teaspoons ground ginger
½ teaspoon ground cloves
¼ teaspoon black pepper

Nightshade free
Gluten free
Lactose free

KALE WITH RAISINS AND TOASTED PINE NUTS

This recipe was originally presented in *Greens, Glorious Greens,* and is shared by my friend, Patrice. The combinations found in this recipe provide a delicious way to enjoy nightshade, gluten, and lactose free cuisine. Serve this recipe over pasta for an exceptional main course. Note: Toast a couple cups of pine nuts, and store in the freezer for many uses later.

Preheat oven to 325 degrees. Serves 2-3.

¼ cup toasted pine nuts
2 cups water
¾ lb. kale, about 6 cups roughly chopped (rinsed and stems removed)
2-3 teaspoons olive oil
2-3 garlic cloves, minced
1/3 cup raisins
Kosher salt, to taste
Black pepper, if desired

Toast pine nuts in oven for 5 minutes, or until golden brown. Be careful not to burn. Set aside. Bring water to a boil in a 10-12 inch skillet with lid. Add prepared kale (as described above). Cook covered, over high heat until tender, about 5 minutes. Drain well and set side. Rinse and dry skillet, heat olive oil over medium heat. Add garlic and saute for 8-10 minutes. Add raisins, saute about 1 minute, stirring constantly to prevent burning. Raisins will be glossy and slightly puffed. Add cooked greens, stir to combine and reheat. Season with salt, and pepper, if desired. Garnish with toasted pine nuts, and serve hot.

Nightshade free
Gluten free
Lactose free

SAVORY PASTAS AND GRAINS

SAVORY PASTAS AND GRAINS

The simplicity of pastas and grains provides a luscious base from which to create savory entrees or side dishes. When these versatile foods are combined with fresh vegetables, chicken, fish, beef, or pork, the outcome is lighter, healthier meal choices.

How to prepare old favorite pasta or grain dishes without nightshades, became a concern when I realized I needed to change my diet. Where would I begin, when I typically included tomatoes and peppers (green, red, yellow, or orange) in most of my pasta and grain dishes? Although, as I proceeded with the needed dietary changes, I found that grains and pastas were just as delicious, without nightshades, and substitutes were endless. With a little imagination, and by adding other interesting ingredients to the dishes, the flavors, textures, and colors, once provided by nightshades, weren't missed.

PASTAS

AUTUMN NIGHT PASTA

Serves 4.

8-10 ounces spaghetti, cooked according to package directions (or gluten free pasta, if needed)
1/3 cup olive oil
3 cups mushrooms, sliced
½ cup onion, chopped
5 cloves garlic, minced
1 cup celery, sliced on diagonal

2 ½ cups asparagus, cut in 1 inch pieces
½ cup Kalamata olives, pitted
1 tablespoon dried oregano
1 pound fresh spinach leaves
1 cup Gorgonzola cheese, softened and crumbled
Kosher salt, white and black peppers, to taste

Cook and drain pasta, according to package directions, to al dente, and keep warm. In a large skillet or wok, sauté the mushrooms and onion, in 3-4 tablespoons olive oil, for about 5 minutes. Add garlic, during the last minute. Add celery and asparagus, sautéing for 3 minutes. Add olives and oregano, then the spinach in batches, as you toss. Add additional olive oil, if needed. Toss vegetable mixture, with Gorgonzola, add salt and peppers, to taste. Serve with crusty bread and seasoned olive oil, for dipping.

Nightshade free
Gluten free (use gluten free pasta)
Lactose free (omit cheese)

SUMMER PASTA SALAD

Serves 8-10.

16 oz. penne pasta, or gluten free pasta
(cooked, rinsed in cold water, and drained)
2 cups broccoli, cut in bite size pieces
1 cup carrots, thinly sliced
Bunch of green onions, sliced
1 cup radish, sliced
1 cup asparagus, cut in 1 inch pieces
1 cup mushrooms, sliced
1 cup golden raisins
1 cup almond slivers
1 cup black olives

2 cups feta cheese, crumbled
2 tablespoons Italian herb mix
Kosher salt and pepper, to taste

Mix all ingredients well, toss with a favorite salad dressing, or the following simple vinaigrette.

VINAIGRETTE
1 cup olive oil
½ cup red wine vinegar
1 tablespoon Dijon mustard
1 teaspoon turmeric
Kosher salt and black pepper, to taste

Whisk ingredients well, pour over pasta salad. Toss gently to mix, refrigerate 1 hour, or until ready to serve. Add extra olive oil, to finish, if desired.

Nightshade free
Gluten free (use gluten free pasta)

ANGEL HAIR PASTA WITH TWO CHEESES

Serves 2

2 - 2 ½ cups young green beans, lightly steamed, cut in 2 inch pieces
6 oz. angel hair pasta, cooked and drained (or gluten free pasta)
2 tablespoons olive oil or butter
2 cups (total) half and half & 1 % milk mix
½ cup cheddar cheese, grated
½ cup mozzarella cheese, grated
Salt and white pepper, to taste
2 tablespoons fresh parsley, minced (garnish)

Keep green beans and pasta warm, while sauce is prepared. Place butter or olive oil, in a small skillet. Heat, then add milk mix. Bring milk to almost boiling, slowly add cheeses, stirring to melt and thicken. Season with salt and pepper. Toss angel hair with cheese sauce and green beans. Serve with a sprinkle of parsley.

Nightshade free

Gluten free (use gluten free pasta)

ANGEL HAIR PASTA WITH VEGETABLE MEDLEY

Serves 2.

6 oz. angel hair pasta, cooked and drained
(or gluten free pasta)
3-4 tablespoons olive oil
4 cups fresh vegetable mix
(such as mushrooms, onions, broccoli, celery, cauliflower, turnips, carrots, garlic, etc.)
2 teaspoons Italian herb mix
3 tablespoons tamari
Kosher salt and pepper, to taste
1 tablespoon preserved lemon, minced (or fresh lemon juice)
½ cup feta cheese

As vegetables and seasonings are prepared, keep cooked pasta warm. Heat olive oil in a large skillet, with lid. Add the vegetable medley with herb mix, tamari, salt, pepper, and preserved lemon. At medium high heat, toss vegetables, until tender crisp. Add additional olive oil, if necessary. Add cheese, toss and cover for 2 minutes, to slightly melt cheese. Mix with warm pasta and serve. Garnish with additional feta cheese, if desired.

Nightshade free

Gluten free (use gluten free pasta)

Lactose free (omit cheese)

TORTELLINI IN ALFREDO SAUCE

Serves 2.

2 cups tortellini, cooked according to package directions
2 tablespoons butter
2 cups half and half (or fat free half and half)
¼ teaspoon white pepper, or to taste
1/8 teaspoon nutmeg
Pinch of salt
1/2 cup Parmesan cheese, and additional for garnish
2 teaspoons fresh parsley, minced

Keep tortellini warm, while making sauce. In a medium skillet, melt butter, add half and half. Add pepper, nutmeg, and pinch of salt. Cook over medium low heat, stirring until sauce slightly thickens, or to desired consistency. Reduce to simmer. Add Parmesan cheese and 1 teaspoon parsley, whisk until smooth. Gently mix well drained tortellini with sauce. Serve in shallow bowls, garnishing with additional Parmesan and parsley.

Nightshade free

CURLY PASTA WITH ARTICHOKES AND SARDINES

Serves 2.

½ (16 oz.) package curly pasta (enhanced with herb flavoring)
Olive oil
1 small white onion, thinly sliced
1 ½ ribs celery, chopped
2 cups oil packed artichokes, halved if large, drained well
¾ cup Kalamata olives, whole and pitted
Salt and pepper, to taste
1 teaspoon garlic flakes
1 tablespoon dried oregano

¾ cup Parmesan cheese
1 tin high quality sardines, drain well (garnish)

Cook curly pasta according to package directions, drain and keep warm. In a medium skillet, add 2-3 tablespoons olive oil, with onion and celery. Saute on high until golden brown, 2-3 minutes. Add artichokes and olives to skillet, with additional olive oil, if needed. Heat, until ingredients sizzle. Add salt and pepper, to taste, garlic flakes, and oregano, mixing well. Gently toss with pasta, splash of olive oil, and Parmesan cheese. Plate, and garnish each dish with 3-4 whole sardines.

Nightshade free

SHRIMP WITH ROSEMARY GARLIC PASTA

Serves 2.

8 tiger shrimp
1/3 cup olive oil
1 teaspoon garlic flakes
1 teaspoon dried basil
1 teaspoon dried oregano, or Italian herb mix
1 teaspoon dill weed
Salt and pepper, to taste
Juice of ½ lemon
½ (8oz.) package curly pasta (enhanced with herb flavoring)
½ small onion, minced
1 ½ ribs celery, minced
½ cup red wine
½ cup cilantro, chopped

Marinate shrimp in olive oil, garlic, basil, oregano, dill weed, salt, pepper, and lemon juice. Refrigerate for 30-45 minutes. Set out 15 minutes prior to cooking. Prepare pasta according to package directions, drain well, and keep warm. Pour shrimp mixture, onion, and celery into *dry* hot skillet, saute for

2-3 minutes. When shrimp is turning pink, add ½ cup red wine, mix well as mixture bubbles. Remove from heat. Splash with a drizzle of olive oil, if needed. Divide pasta between two serving plates, add half the cilantro to each serving, followed by half the shrimp mixture. Serve immediately.
Nightshade and lactose free

BLUE CHEESE AND SPINACH WITH SPAGHETTI

Serves 2-3.

Spaghetti for 2-3 servings (gluten free, if desired)
1 cup half and half
1 cup 2 % milk
¾ cup crumbled blue cheese
2 tablespoons fresh onion, minced
1 teaspoon dried tarragon
Salt and pepper, to taste
4 cups fresh spinach, packed down
1 tablespoon (each) water and butter
Sliced radish and parsley, garnish

Prepare spaghetti, following package directions. Drain and keep warm. **For sauce:** In a small pan over medium heat, combine half and half, milk, blue cheese, onion, tarragon, with salt and pepper, to taste. As sauce warms and cheese begins to melt, reduce heat to simmer. Stir often, as sauce thickens. Set aside. **For spinach:** In a medium skillet over medium high heat, place spinach with water and butter, cover. When spinach begins to steam and wilt, remove lid, stir to evaporate moisture, or blot bottom of pan with paper towel. **To assemble:** Gently toss spaghetti, sauce, and spinach, just before serving. Garnish with sliced radish and parsley sprig.
Nightshade free
Gluten free (use gluten free pasta)

SPAGHETTI WITH LEMON, GARLIC, AND BACON

Serves 2.

6-8 oz. spaghetti, cooked, drained, and keep warm
4 sliced bacon, fried and crumbled
3 tablespoons olive oil (more for finish)
4 large garlic cloves, minced
2 tablespoons preserved lemon, minced
1 tablespoon dried basil
3 tablespoons chives, sliced in ½ inch pieces
½ cup Parmesan or Romano cheese

In a small skillet, add olive oil with garlic, lemon, and basil. Saute 3-4 minutes. Combine with cooked spaghetti, bacon, and chives. Drizzle additional olive oil, if needed, toss with cheese.

Nightshade free
Lactose free

GRAINS

QUINOA SALAD

A wonderful summer luncheon entrée for the patio or picnic in the country. Preheat oven to 375 degrees. Serves 3-4.

2 large carrots, thinly sliced
2 large beets, peeled and diced
6 cloves garlic, whole
2 cups cooked quinoa, set aside
2-3 cups arugula, rinsed and dried
2 cans white kidney beans, rinsed and drained

1- 1 ½ cups grilled chicken, lamb, or shrimp,
seasoned well and diced (optional)
Salt and pepper, to taste

Toss carrots, beets, and garlic in olive oil, roast at 375 degrees, for approximately 30 minutes, or until tender and slightly crisp. Cool, mix with other ingredients. (Chicken, lamb, or shrimp are optional.) When ready to serve, toss with desired amount of vinaigrette below, or other favorite dressing.

VINIAGRETTE
¾ cup olive oil
¼ cup fresh lemon juice
1 teaspoon oregano, dried
Salt, white and black peppers, to taste

Nightshade free
Gluten free
Lactose free

QUINOA WITH APRICOTS AND GOLDEN RAISINS

This fragrant, but simple side dish is perfect with Moroccan foods, pork tenderloin, or ham. Other dried fruits, such as prunes and cherries, are good additions to this savory selection as well. Serves 6-8.

1 cup quinoa, cooked according to package directions
¾ cup dried apricots, chopped
¾ cup golden raisins

While quinoa is cooking, add fruits. Cook covered, approximately 12-15 minutes, or until water is absorbed. Set aside covered, for at least 15 minutes before serving. Can be served warm, or at room temperature.

Nightshade free
Gluten free
Lactose free

CORN RICE CHEESE BAKE

This amazing casserole, adapted from a *Colorado Cache* recipe, is a hit every time. Minor adjustments eliminated the nightshades, without compromising the flavor. Serve at a dinner buffet, casual barbeque, or any holiday occasion. Freezes well. Preheat oven to 300 degrees. Serves 8.

1 cup white rice, cooked
2 cups celery, chopped
4 tablespoons onion, chopped
1/3 cup butter
3 ½ cups frozen corn
3 cups (total) grated cheddar and Monterey Jack mix
1 ½ cups milk
1 teaspoon salt
½ - 1 teaspoon white pepper
Vegetable oil spray

Cook rice, making 3 cups fluffy white rice. (Recommend using Calrose rice.) Set aside. Sauté celery and onion in butter for about 5 -7 minutes. Mix with remaining ingredients, tossing well. Place in a 2 quart casserole, coated with vegetable oil spray. Cover tightly and bake in a 300 degree preheated oven for 1 hour, or until center is hot and slightly bubbly.

Nightshade free
Gluten free

PECAN WILD RICE

My daughter, Kelli and family, enjoy this recipe during the holidays. It's a lovely alternative to other grains, and adds pizzazz to a festive gathering. Serves 6.

5 ½ cups chicken stock
1 cup wild rice, uncooked
4 green onions, thinly sliced

1 cup pecan halves, toasted
1 cup golden raisins
1/3 cup orange juice
¼ cup parsley, minced
¼ cup olive oil
1 tablespoon orange rind zest
1 ½ teaspoon Kosher salt
¼ teaspoon coarse black pepper

Combine stock and rice in a medium sauce pan. Bring to boil, reduce heat. Simmer rice uncovered for 45 minutes, or until rice is done. Drain and place in a medium bowl. While rice is hot, add remaining ingredients, toss gently. Adjust seasonings. Serve immediately.

Nightshade free
Gluten free
Lactose free

SAVORY OATMEAL WITH EGG AND SPINACH

Something for a special and different Sunday morning breakfast.
Serves 2-4 servings.

1 cup oatmeal
1 ¾ cups water
3-4 teaspoons butter
1 teaspoon oregano, dried
Salt and black pepper, to taste
½ cup ham, minced
1/3 cup light cream cheese
Vegetable oil spray
½ cup mushrooms, minced
½ cup celery, minced

1/3 cup onion, minced
1/8 teaspoon garlic flakes
2 teaspoons water
3 cups fresh spinach, packed
4-8 eggs, depending on servings (two per person)

Prepare oatmeal, with water, according to directions on package. Add 2-3 teaspoons of butter, oregano, salt, and pepper, while oats cook. When done, stir in chopped ham and cream cheese, blending well. Set aside and keep warm. Place mushrooms, celery, and onion, in a large skillet, coated with vegetable oil spray. Cook until slightly browned. Add garlic flakes, water, spinach, and 1 teaspoon butter, to the skillet. Toss to wilt. (Blot spinach with paper towel, to remove any moisture remaining in skillet.) Prepare eggs, as desired.

To assemble the dish: Place serving of oatmeal mixture in bottom of medium, shallow bowls. Add spinach and vegetable mixture in the center of each portion, followed by serving of eggs.

Nightshade free
Gluten free

CAROLINE'S OAT AND OAT BRAN MUFFINS

Oat bran muffins were first popular, in the late 1980s. These muffins are high in fiber, great at breakfast, or on a hike. Makes 14-16 muffins.

Preheat oven to 425 degrees.

Blend dry ingredients:
2 ½ cups oat bran cereal
2 cups old fashioned oats
1 teaspoon baking powder
½ teaspoon salt
2 teaspoon ground ginger
½ teaspoon nutmeg

1 teaspoon ground cinnamon
1 to 1½ cups golden raisins

Whisk the following liquid ingredients:
4-6 tablespoons agave, to taste (or honey)
2 eggs, beaten
1 cup canola oil
1 ½ cups 1% milk

Coat muffin tins with vegetable oil spray. Blend the dry and liquid ingredients. Fill each muffin cup ¾ full. Bake for 15-18 minutes. **Cool before removing from pan**. Muffins freeze well. Tasty additions for the muffins are: Pecans, walnuts, or dried fruits such as chopped prunes, cherries, apricots, or apples.
Nightshade free
(Gluten research is unclear as to oats or oat bran.)

BASIC ITALIAN POLENTA

This traditional recipe is for sliced polenta, which has numerous uses. Serve with tapenade, pesto, steamed vegetables, or savory sauces. For smooth polenta, or one that is more fluid, reduce cooking time. Serves 6-8.

6 cups water
About 1 teaspoon salt
2 cups polenta (corn grits)
3 tablespoons butter
Grated or shredded cheese, such as:
Parmesan, Romano, fontina, or Monterey Jack

In a deep pan over high heat, bring water and ½ teaspoon salt, to a boil. Gradually add polenta, stirring constantly. Reduce heat, simmer gently to prevent sticking until mixture thickens, about 25-30 minutes, or until very thick. Continue to stir, until done. Add cheese and blend well. Adjust salt. Spoon polenta into a glass container coated with vegetable oil spray. Spread evenly, to cool. When ready to serve, turn polenta onto a flat surface and slice. (Please read directions on polenta package, for additional instructions. Products may slightly vary. Quick cooking polenta is also available.) Serve with eggs, grilled chicken, pork, fish, or roasted vegetables.

Nightshade free

Gluten free

CHEESE GRITS FOR MANY USES

This basic recipe for cheese grits is as versatile as any pasta. It's a wonderful addition at breakfast or brunch, but is also a companion for seafood, pork, or vegetarian dishes. Different cheeses can be interchanged with the recipe, along with herbs, dried or fresh. Please see recipe for *Shrimp Towers,* in chapter *Fish and Seafood to Delight,* as a variation. Serves 4-5 as a side dish, or as a layer in a *tower.*

3 cups water
½ teaspoon salt
Black pepper, to taste
½ teaspoon garlic flakes
1 tablespoon dried oregano
½ tablespoon dried thyme
1 tablespoon butter
¾ cup corn grits
Parmesan, goat, cheddar, fontina, or Monterey Jack cheeses

Bring water, salt, pepper, garlic, herbs, and butter to boil, add grits slowly. Reduce heat to simmer, cooking approximately 5 minutes, until thick and creamy. While cooking, partially cover to prevent splatters or burns. When grits are done, add a favorite cheese, and blend well. For a creamier consistency, whisk to finish.

Nightshade free

Gluten free

EGGS FOR EVERY OCCASION

EGGS FOR EVERY OCCASION

Eggs may be the most underrated food we use today. At brunch or luncheon, egg casseroles or stratas become center stage, but there are hundreds of other uses. The options are endless, and of course, eggs are nightshade, gluten, and lactose free.

EGGS WITH WASABI GUACAMOLE

Guacamole prepared with wasabi is a lovely addition to the egg dish below. The recipe for spicy, nightshade free *Guacamole with Wasabi,* is found in *Appetizers for Festive Starts.* Prepare 1/3 cup guacamole for each serving. Recipe below serves 4.

Vegetable oil spray
3-4 tablespoon olive oil
1 cup onion, minced
12 eggs (3 per person)
Kosher salt and pepper, to taste
Lime wedges, cilantro, and radish, for garnish

Coat medium skillet with vegetable oil spray and olive oil. Quickly sear minced onion. Add eggs that have been whisked with salt and pepper.
Cook, until fluffy, but not dry. Plate eggs, top with guacamole. Garnish with lime wedge, cilantro, and radish slices.

Nightshade free
Gluten free
Lactose free

EGGS WITH DILL, TRUFFLE OIL, AND ARUGULA

This egg dish, prepared in three easy steps, is perfect for special breakfasts or your next brunch. The flavors are complex, but come together magically. Serves 2.

5 eggs
½ teaspoon white pepper
½ teaspoon salt
½ teaspoon dill weed
Vegetable oil spray
3-4 tablespoons olive oil
½ cup onion, coarsely chopped
½ cup broccoli, cut into small pieces
10 black olives, sliced

Whisk eggs, white pepper, salt, and dill weed, set aside. Heavily spray medium size skillet with vegetable oil spray, add olive oil. Place onion, broccoli, and olives, in skillet and saute until vegetables are tender crisp. Pour egg mixture into skillet, gently stir with a lifting motion, until eggs are set, but not dry. Cover with a clean towel, to keep warm. Prepare the following.

3 cups arugula, rinsed and dried
2 tablespoons olive oil
Salt and black pepper
4 tablespoons Parmesan cheese
Truffle oil
3-4 strawberries

Toss arugula, olive oil, salt, pepper, and Parmesan, divide on two plates. Add serving of eggs in center of salads. Drizzle eggs lightly with truffle oil. Garnish with sliced strawberries. Serve immediately.

Nightshade free
Gluten free
Lactose free (omit cheese)

STEAM FRIED EGGS

A very simple way to prepare eggs that brings out the flavor. Serves 1.

Vegetable oil spray
1 teaspoon olive oil
2 whole eggs
Kosher salt and pepper, to taste
Fresh basil or other fresh herb (optional)

In a small skillet with lid, heavily coat bottom with vegetable oil spray, add olive oil. Place skillet on high heat for one minute, add 2 eggs. Lightly season with salt and black pepper. If desired, add 1-2 tablespoons fresh basil, thinly sliced, or other favorite fresh herb. When eggs begin to set, reduce heat to medium low, cover skillet. Cook eggs 2-4 minutes, as desired. Do not turn. Eggs can be cooked by this method *sunny side up* to *hard.* This style of cooking eggs can be used in many of the recipes found in this section.

Nightshade free
Gluten free
Lactose free

CREAMED SPINACH NESTS WITH EGGS AND POLENTA

This recipe was inspired by a Rachel Ray recipe, in 2011. I've modified the ingredients to eliminate nightshades, and have added a layer of polenta which enhances the casserole. Preheat oven to 400 degrees. Serves 6-8.

The Polenta:
6 cups water
1/2 teaspoon salt
2 cups polenta corn grits
3 tablespoons butter
Grated or shredded cheese such as:
Parmesan, Romano, fontina, or Monterey Jack

In a medium deep pan over high heat, bring water and salt to a boil. Gradually add polenta, continuously stirring. Reduce heat, simmering gently to prevent sticking until mixture thickens, about 15-20 minutes. Continue to stir. Add cheese, as desired. For this application, polenta should be spreadable and thick, but not stiff. When polenta is ready, spread mixture in the bottom of a large casserole, coated with vegetable oil spray. Set aside.

The Eggs and Spinach Nests:
¼ stick butter
½ onion, chopped
2 pounds spinach leaves
Salt and white pepper
½ teaspoon garlic flakes
½ teaspoon nutmeg
½ cup half and half
Vegetable oil spray
6-8 eggs (one per nest)
3/4 cup Parmesan cheese
Bacon strips, fried crisp (optional)

In a large skillet, melt butter, and saute onion, until translucent. Add spinach in batches to steam, using tongs. If moisture remains in skillet when spinach is done, use paper towels to absorb. Season with salt and pepper, to taste, garlic flakes, and nutmeg. Mix well. Add half and half, simmering until slightly thickened, approximately 2 minutes. Adjust seasonings. Arrange the spinach mixture into 6-8 *nests* (or small wells), on the polenta base. Fill each *nest* with a raw egg and 1-2 tablespoons of Parmesan. Bake uncovered in oven for 10-12 minutes, until egg whites are set, but yokes are slightly runny. Add fried bacon strips, if desired.

Nightshade free
Gluten free

EGGS AND ARTICHOKE TOWERS

Prepare one recipe of Cheese Grits, as described in *Savory Pastas and Grains.* Set aside and keep warm. Serves 4.

3/4 cup celery, chopped
3/4 cup onion, minced
2 tablespoons butter
2 cups oil packed artichoke hearts, well drained
8 eggs, cooked as preferred
Fresh fruits, for garnish

In a medium skillet, combine celery, onion, and butter. Sauté until tender crisp. Fold in artichoke hearts and heat thoroughly. Place serving of *Cheese Grits* in center of each plate, forming a well. Top with a serving of artichoke mixture, followed by a portion of the eggs, to form tower. Garnish with fresh raspberries, or other colorful fruit.

Nightshade free
Gluten free

EGG, BLACK OLIVE, AND ONION PIE

Preheat broiler to high heat. Serves 8.

12 eggs, whisk until smooth, set aside
4 large sweet onions, chopped, or very thinly sliced
3 - 4 tablespoons olive oil
½ cup Madeira sherry
1 cup black olives, sliced
1 teaspoon oregano
1 teaspoon thyme
½ teaspoon nutmeg
Salt and black pepper, to taste
1 cup Parmesan cheese

In 15” oven proof skillet, sauté onions in olive oil, until translucent. Add Madeira, olives, oregano, thyme, nutmeg, salt and pepper, mixing well. Raise heat to high, to reduce liquids to ½ cup, and continue cooking. Turn heat to medium, pour eggs over onion mixture. Do not stir, at this point. Sprinkle Parmesan cheese over top of egg pie, cover. When eggs begin to set, remove lid, and place under preheated broiler for approximately 10-15 minutes, or until done. Remove when eggs are completely set, but not dry. Test with dry toothpick. Let stand 10 minutes, before cutting into wedges or squares.

Nightshade free
Gluten free
Lactose free (omit cheese)

LEFTOVER SALMON, MUSHROOMS, AND EGGS

When I grill salmon, I save 4-5 ounces of the cooked fish, for something special the following day. Prepare this simple recipe for a casual supper, served with a crisp green salad. Serves 2-3.

5-6 eggs, whisk with salt and pepper, to taste
Vegetable oil spray
1-2 tablespoons olive oil
3 cups mushrooms, sliced
1 ½ cups onion, coarsely chopped
Kosher salt and pepper, to taste
4-5 ounces grilled, seasoned salmon
Truffle oil

Whisk eggs, set aside. In a medium skillet coated with vegetable oil spray, over medium high heat, add olive oil, mushrooms, and onion. Saute until most of the water has been released and evaporated from the mushrooms. Lightly season with salt and pepper. Tear grilled salmon into small pieces, add to mushroom mixture, combine quickly. Pour eggs over skillet ingredients, scramble until set, but not dry. Plate, drizzle with truffle oil.

Nightshade free
Gluten and lactose free

ASPARAGUS AND BLACK OLIVE FRITTATA

Preheat broiler to high. Serves 6.

12 eggs, beaten
1 tablespoon dried tarragon
Salt and white pepper, to taste
Vegetable oil spray
3-4 tablespoons olive oil
½ onion, chopped
6-8 mushrooms, sliced
1 cup black olives, coarsely chopped
6-8 stems asparagus, trimmed and cut in 1 inch pieces
2 tablespoons capers, optional
1 cup Parmesan cheese, or other favorite choice

To beaten eggs, add tarragon, salt and white pepper, to taste. Set aside. Coat medium oven proof skillet with vegetable oil spray and 3-4 tablespoons olive oil. Saute onion, mushrooms, and olives, for 4-5 minutes. During last 2 minutes, add asparagus and capers. Over medium heat, add egg mixture and cheese. Do not stir. Cover skillet for approximately 3-4 minutes, to begin setting eggs. When eggs *bubble around edges* of pan, remove lid, place under preheated broiler for about 5-8 minutes, to finish cooking process. For doneness, check with a dry toothpick. Let stand 5 minutes before serving.

Nightshade free
Gluten free
Lactose free (omit cheese)

SPINACH ORZO SQUARES

This casserole has been in our family, since the 1970s, but remains a favorite for brunches, holiday breakfasts, pot lucks, etc.

Preheat oven to 375 degrees. Serves 8-10.

Vegetable oil spray
16-18 ounces of frozen chopped spinach or
frozen chopped collard greens (thaw and squeeze dry)
12-14 eggs, beaten
2 cups mushrooms, minced and microwave
with 1 tablespoon butter, slightly drained
1 medium onion, chopped and microwave
with 1 tablespoon butter, until tender
1 cup cottage cheese
8 ounces Parmesan
1 stick butter, melted
1 teaspoon nutmeg
1 teaspoon salt
1 teaspoon white pepper
Black pepper, to taste
3 teaspoons Italian dry herb mix, or oregano
1 garlic clove, minced
1-2 cups cooked orzo pasta

Heavily coat an 15x10.5" baking dish with vegetable oil spray. Mix all ingredients except the cooked orzo pasta, blending well. When combined, add cooked pasta, for desired consistency. Fill casserole dish, and bake approximately 1 hour, or until firmly set and slightly browned on top. Let stand 10-15 minutes, before cutting in squares. Serve warm.

Nightshade free

TARRAGON AND TURMERIC EGGS

Serves 2.

5 eggs, beaten
½ teaspoon ground turmeric
½ - 3/4 teaspoon dried tarragon
Vegetable oil spray
3 tablespoons olive oil
5 mushrooms, sliced
½ sweet onion, coarsely chopped
Salt and pepper
½ cup cilantro, chopped
Whole wheat toast
Truffle oil

To beaten eggs, add turmeric and tarragon, whisk and set aside. In a medium skillet coated with vegetable oil spray, add 2-3 tablespoons olive oil, mushrooms, onion, with salt and pepper, to taste. Saute until vegetables are tender crisp, and moisture evaporates. Add eggs, tossing gently to cook. When eggs are beginning to set, add cilantro, to finish. Plate eggs over whole wheat toast. Lightly drizzle eggs with truffle oil. Serve immediately.

Nightshade free
Gluten free (use gluten free bread for toast)
Lactose free

EGG AND QUINOA STIR-FRY

Serves 1 main course, or 2 side dishes.

Vegetable oil spray
1 tablespoon olive oil
2 mushrooms, sliced
½ cup carrot, thinly sliced
1/3 cup onion, chopped

½ cup fresh asparagus, in 1 inch slices
2 eggs, beaten
¼ teaspoon turmeric
Kosher salt and pepper, to taste
¾ cup cooked quinoa
Tamari
2-3 cooked shrimp, chopped (optional)

Coat small skillet with vegetable oil spray, add olive oil. Add mushrooms, carrots, and onion, then stir-fry for 3 minutes. Add asparagus, stir-fry 1 minute more. Pour beaten eggs over vegetables, and sprinkle with seasonings. Stir egg mixture to begin cooking process, add quinoa, as eggs begin to set. Continue stirring to blend ingredients and flavors. As an option, add cooked, diced shrimp, just before serving. Pass tamari at table.

Nightshade free
Gluten free
Lactose free

CAROLINE'S DEVILED EGGS...TWO WAYS

This recipe is found in *Appetizers for Festive Starts.* If you like anchovies, you'll like this recipe. They are delicious as appetizers at cocktail parties, but they are a nice addition for holiday buffets and picnics.

VEGETABLE QUICHE, WITH MANY OPTIONS

The following recipe offers many different ways to prepare and enjoy quiche, using this basic egg filling. Vegetables, cheeses, and other ingredients can be changed, as preferred. Each quiche serves 6-8.

BASIC EGG FILLING
6 eggs
1 cup 2 % lactose free milk

1-2 teaspoon salt
1 teaspoon black pepper
3 heaping tablespoons flour
(Herb options: dill weed, tarragon, nutmeg, etc.)

Beat eggs well, add milk, salt and pepper. Whisk, while adding flour slowly, to blend any lumps. When smooth, set aside.

BASIC CRUST (for 9" pie plate)
½ cup white flour
½ cup whole wheat flour
1/3 cup cold butter
3 tablespoons cold water

With pastry cutter or fork, blend flours and butter. When uniformly blended, and mixture is mealy, add about 3 tablespoons cold water. Mix well, gently with hands, chill 1 hour. When ready, roll out dough, place in pie plate. Trim dough, pinch edges. Set aside. (Quiche can be prepared "crustless," but oil and/or butter pie pan well, when using this method. You may also use commercial refrigerated crusts.)

SAUTE FOR BASIC VEGETABLES
1 medium onion, minced
12 mushrooms, sliced or chopped
2 teaspoon butter
1 teaspoon olive oil

(Vegetable and other ingredient options: Spinach, broccoli, asparagus, artichoke hearts, green onion, olives, capers, etc.)

In medium skillet, add onion and mushrooms, with butter and olive oil. Saute until tender. You may add other vegetables, olives, etc. at this point, if desired. Set aside.

CHEESE FOR QUICHE
Almost any type of grated cheese works well with quiche.

Place about 1 cup of cheese in bottom of pan over crust, add half the sautéed vegetable mix. Add a second cup of cheese, followed by remainder of vegetable mix.

ASSEMBLY:

When crust is in pie pan, and vegetables and cheese have been added, gently pour egg mixture over contents. Place pie plate on a cookie sheet, lined with foil. Bake in preheated oven at 375 degrees for 45 minutes. During the last 10 minutes, raise heat to 400 degrees. To check doneness, test center of quiche with toothpick. Set on baking rack to cool for 15-20 minutes, before serving.

Nightshade free

Gluten free (when prepared crustless)

EGG CASSEROLE FOR A SPECIAL BRUNCH

My friend, Pat, from Oklahoma City, served this fabulous dish at a brunch she hosted for friends while I was visiting. It was a treat then, and it will be a treat at your next brunch. Serves 18-20.

2 cans undiluted mushroom soup
¼ cup sherry
Kosher salt and pepper, to taste
1 can sliced water chestnuts, drained
1 can sliced mushrooms, drained
1 can mushroom caps, drained
1 stick butter
½ cup milk
3 dozen eggs, beaten
½ lb. sharp cheddar, grated

Over medium heat, melt undiluted soup, with sherry, salt, and pepper. Add water chestnuts, mushroom slices and mushroom caps, set aside. In a very large skillet, melt butter. Whisk milk and eggs together, place in skillet and soft scramble, set aside. In a 15x11 inch buttered casserole, layer ½ the scrambled eggs, followed by half the soup/mushroom mixture, and half the grated cheese. Repeat for a second layer. Refrigerate overnight. Bring to room temperature, bake at 300-325 degrees in a preheated oven for 1 hour, or until bubbly hot. If desired, place under broiler for a couple minutes, to brown.

Nightshade free

Gluten free

SURPRISING PIZZAS

SURPRISING PIZZAS

It may be difficult to imagine pizza without tomatoes, peppers, and spicy tomato sauces, but try one of the nightshade free pizza recipes below, for a pleasant surprise. This is pizza you can get excited about, and pizza your guests will enjoy as well.

I recommend using fresh focaccia bread dough for the base of my pizzas, although there are several options that you may want to try. Whole wheat tortillas, commercial non-frozen or frozen pizza crusts are available in most supermarkets. If you're a baker, there are numerous recipes for pizza crust.

For gluten free pizzas, use gluten free crusts which are also available in most markets.

At some supermarkets, you can purchase fresh focaccia bread dough, in the bakery areas. Twelve ounces of this luscious dough makes a perfectly sized pizza crust. Simply, roll out the dough on a floured surface, then place on a cookie sheet and top with your favorite ingredients. The raw dough freezes well. Keep several in your freezer, for convenience.

Pizza toppings are endless. While in Italy, back in the 1970s, I had pizza that had corn and green peas as part of the topping. It seemed strange at the time, but recently, I had pizza at a local high-end pizzeria, which featured corn suspended in a delightful, smooth cheese base. So much for stereotypes. For lactose free pizzas, omit cheeses.

In this section, the focus is no nightshades, but as I mentioned, these pizzas can be enjoyed by everyone. The recipes are simple, and take *little time* to prepare. Included below is a recipe that can be used as a template for creating your own pizzas. There are also suggestions for ingredients that you may wish to try. Please don't miss the *breakfast pizza.*

SPINACH, MUSHROOM, AND TWO CHEESE PIZZA

Preheat oven to 400 degrees. Serves 2-4 as entrée, or 10 as appetizer, cut into small squares.

12 oz. focaccia bread dough
(purchased at supermarket bakery, or other crust)
Flour
Vegetable oil spray
Olive oil
Kosher salt and black pepper
Garlic flakes
Oregano
White pepper (optional)
3 cups fresh spinach
2 cups, mushrooms, thinly sliced
¾ cup black olives, sliced
1 ½ cups mozzarella cheese
½ cup feta, crumbled

On a flour prepared flat surface, roll out the focaccia bread dough to ¼-½ inch thickness. (Flour top of the dough as well as the rolling pin. A clean wine bottle may substitute as a rolling pin.) When shaped and smooth, fold dough in half and transfer to a cookie sheet coated with vegetable oil spray. Thinly spread olive oil over the entire top surface. Season with salt, black pepper, garlic flakes, and dried oregano. For an added *spicy* option, also season with white pepper, if desired. Layer spinach over the dough, about 1 ½ inches high. Add mushrooms and black olives. Top with mozzarella and feta cheeses. Sprinkle lightly again with salt, black pepper, garlic flakes, and oregano. Bake at 400 degrees for approximately 18-19 minutes, or until edges of crust and cheeses have slightly browned.

CREATE YOUR OWN PIZZA FAVORITES

Using the pizza concept as described in the above recipe, you can serve delicious hot pizzas to your friends or family in about 30 minutes, start to finish. Mix and match the ingredients, as you choose, and include your favorites, as well. For starters, the following suggestions may be helpful.

PIZZA CRUST OPTIONS

1. **Fresh focaccia bread dough (purchased or home made)**
2. **Whole wheat tortillas**
3. **Gluten free crusts**
4. **Commercial frozen or non-frozen pizza crusts**
5. **Flatbread**
6. **Other commercial crusts**

BASE AND SEASONINGS (first ingredients on crust)

Spread one of the following ingredients over the pizza crust, season as you desire with salt, white or black pepper, garlic flakes, and dried or fresh herbs.

1. **Olive oil, or flavored enhanced olive oil**
2. **Basil pesto**
3. **Toasted walnut pesto**
4. **Mushroom pesto**
5. **Lemon and garlic hummus**
6. **Tapenade**

TOPPINGS

Use three or more of the following ingredients to create an interesting, nightshade free pizza. Mix, match, and experiment.

1. **Almost any cheese, or combination of cheeses**
2. **Pitted and sliced olives of various types (Remember, no pimientos in olives.)**
3. **Capers**
4. **Vegetables: yellow squash, zucchini, all types of mushrooms, green onions, yellow onions, asparagus, broccoli, spinach, kale, whole roasted garlic cloves, marinated artichokes hearts, various beans, etc.**
5. **Sliced, chopped, or roasted: almonds, pine nuts, walnuts, etc.**
6. **Preserved lemon, minced**
7. **Your favorite dried or fresh herbs**
8. **Ham or prosciutto, cooked hamburger, diced cooked chicken, anchovy, etc.**
9. **Pineapple, dried cranberries, etc.**

BREAKFAST PIZZA

For something different at breakfast, try pizza topped with eggs.

1. **Start with an olive oil base, spread over crust.**
2. **Add 2-3 cheeses to the pizza such as cheddar, Parmesan, mozzarella, and Monterey Jack.**
3. **Add herbs and seasonings, of choice.**
4. **Fresh asparagus works well with this pizza.**
5. **When pizza is arranged as you wish, add 4 raw eggs, carefully placed around pizza.**
6. **Sprinkle pizza with fresh parsley and Parmesan cheese.**

7. **Bake in preheated oven of 400 degrees, until eggs are set and crust is slightly browned, about 18-20 minutes.**
8. **Cut into four servings, one egg centering each slice. This pizza makes an interesting presentation, and is a decadent way to begin your day.**

DESSERTS AND OTHER FINE FINISHES

DESSERTS AND OTHER FINE FINISHES

Desserts are favorite finishes at dinner parties and family gatherings. I avoid sugar, so I have developed recipes that provide a bit of sweet at the end of the meal, but at the same time, are basically sugar free or have a minimal amount of sugar. I use agave as a sugar substitute for many of my recipes, although honey may be substituted.

POACHED PEARS WITH CRANBERRY GINGER TOPPINIG

Serves 6.

PEARS
6 firm, ripe pears, whole
1 cup white wine, such as a chardonnay
1 ½ cup water
½ cup agave, or to taste
Cinnamon stick
¼ teaspoon ground cloves
2 tablespoons butter

Wash pears, and leave stems intact. Place pears lying on their sides in a large, deep skillet, with lid. Add ingredients, cover, and bring to a boil. Reduce to simmer, cook until tender, approximately 12-15 minutes. Turn pears once during simmer. Pears should be tender, but firm. Cool without lid. Refrigerate until serving, or serve at room temperature. Serves 6.

GINGER CRANBERRY TOPPING
12 oz. fresh cranberries, rinsed and drained

1 cup water
3/4 cup agave, or to taste
1 cinnamon stick
2 -3 tablespoons fresh ginger, minced

Combine all ingredients in a small sauce pan, with lid. Heat to bubbling, partially covered to prevent splatters or possible burns. When the cranberries thicken, stir well, and set aside. Cool, refrigerate. When ready to serve, stand one pear in center of dessert plate. Drizzle cranberry topping over pear.

Nightshade free
Gluten free
Lactose free

CHEESE PLATTER WITH FRUITS AND TRUFFLES

1. **On a decorative platter, place two or three favorite cheeses, such as a Gorgonzola, Irish white cheddar, or Brie.**
2. **Let cheese stand to room temperature 1-2 hours, before serving.**
3. **Select 2-3 fruits that are in season, to pair with the cheeses. Strawberries and pears are often a good choices, for color and flavor.**
4. **For a special touch, and for those who enjoy a bit of chocolate, include truffles or other confection.**

Nightshade free
Gluten free

GEORGE'S APPLE PIE WITH AGAVE

Cooking with agave, to replace sugar, has become a habit at our house. This pie was created to provide guests with a dessert that is sugar free, but at the same time, delicious. George did the test recipe for this lovely pie, and of course, he got the first piece. Other fruits can be substituted for the apples, as variations on this recipe. Preheat oven to 400 degrees, and place rack in bottom 1/3 of oven. Serves 6-8.

2 commercially prepared pie crusts
Vegetable oil spray
5 medium apples, UNPEELED and sliced
2 teaspoons fresh lemon juice
¾ cup agave
3 tablespoons cornstarch
1 ½ teaspoon cinnamon
¼ teaspoon nutmeg
3-4 tablespoons butter
1 egg white and 1 teaspoon water, beaten (egg wash)

Bring pie crust to room temperature. Coat bottom of a 10 inch pie plate, with vegetable oil spray. Add first piece of pie crust, adjust to bottom of plate, trim edges. Core and slice apples, leaving skin. Toss with lemon juice, set aside. In a separate bowl, combine agave, cornstarch, cinnamon, and nutmeg. Blend well, toss gently with apples. Pour apples into pie shell. Dot pie with butter. Add second piece of pie crust to top, trim edges and crimp. Brush egg wash over top of pie, cut a decorative slit to vent top crust. Lay a piece of foil on second rack beneath pie, to catch any drips as pie bakes. Bake at 400 degrees for approximately 50 minutes, or until golden brown and juices begin to seep thru vent in top of pie. Let stand 3 hours before cutting.

Note: To easily core, stand an apple on cutting board, slice wedges of apple, while circling the core. Slice wedges into thin slices for the pie, and proceed with recipe.

Nightshade free

SLICED NAVAL ORANGES WITH KAILUA

Naval oranges
(approximately ½ - ¾ orange per person,
peeled and left whole)
Raspberries
Kailua liqueur

Slice whole oranges in ½ inch circles, through diameter, arrange on individual dessert plates. Top with raspberries. Drizzle Kailua, over oranges. Let set 10 minutes, before serving.

Nightshade free
Gluten free
Lactose free

BAKED APPLES IN DUBONNET

Preheat oven to 350 degrees. Serves 4

4 Gala apples (or other favorite),
cored and leave bottom intact
3 tablespoons dried cranberries
2 tablespoons golden raisins
2 tablespoons sliced almonds
½ teaspoon cinnamon
2 tablespoons agave (or honey)
½ cup Dubonnet, plus extra
2 teaspoons butter

Prep apples, set aside. Mix cranberries, raisins, almonds, cinnamon, and agave with ½ cup Dubonnet, let stand for 1 hour. Place cored apples, standing up, in a shallow baking dish lined with foil. Fill cores with fruit mixture, arrange extra filling on top of each apple. Press to secure. Carefully drizzle additional Dubonnet over apples. Dot each apple with ½ teaspoon butter.

Add ½ cup water in bottom of baking dish. Bake for approximately 25-30 minutes, or until apples are tender. Serve warm or at room temperature.
Nightshade free
Gluten and lactose free

STRAWBERRIES WITH FRESH LIME AND CINNAMON

Serves 4

2 tablespoons agave
1 tablespoon butter
2 tablespoons fresh lime juice
¼ teaspoon cinnamon
2 cups fresh strawberries, quartered
Greek yogurt, optional

In a medium skillet over medium heat, combine first 4 ingredients. Cook until slightly thickened. Add strawberries and toss, for 2 minutes. Serve immediately over Greek yogurt, slightly sweetened with agave, if desired.
Nightshade free
Gluten free

BRIE AND BISCOTTI

Brie
Agave
1 small apple, diced (or other fruit, diced)
Biscotti or shortbread

Shave the top of Brie gently, discard. Top with apple, or other fruit, then drizzle agave over cheese, to adequately cover. Just before serving, heat in microwave, until warm. Honey can replace agave, if desired. Pass biscotti,

shortbread, or ginger snaps/wafer. Serves 6-8. Note: See *Pennyquick Shortbread* recipe below.
Nightshade free

MINTED GRAPEFRUIT

Grapefruit sections, 3-4 per person (from jar or fresh)
Triple Sec
Fresh mint
Strawberry slices, garnish

Arrange grapefruit sections on dessert plates or in martini glasses. Drizzle triple sec over fruit. Garnish with mint and strawberry slices.
Nightshade free
Gluten free
Lactose free

PENNYQUICK SHORTBREAD AND FIVE GENERATIONS

This historic family recipe was given to me by my friend, Nan, who has brought this delightful dessert to many parties at my home over the years. For five generations, the women in Nan's family have made this shortbread recipe. Lovingly, I include the history of this recipe. Preheat oven to 325 degrees. Serves 10-16.

2 cups flour, sifted
½ cup sugar
½ lb. butter, softened

Mix ingredients and work well with hands until dough is uniform and forms a nice ball. Divide dough in half and pat down firmly, in the bottom of two 9" metal pie pans. Made radial marks with a fork. Bake for 20-25 minutes, or until edges are barely brown. Remove from oven, *immediately* cut with a sharp knife into 16 pie shaped slices. Leave in pan to cool. Variation: Add bits of candied ginger.

The History:
Five generations of women have made this shortbread. What do I know of them? I know the first one braved the heat of India wearing a corset. I know she kissed her children goodbye (the ones that survived), as they boarded a ship to England. I know one of her daughters came to face the bleak winters and isolation of Wyoming, and raised her family while fiercely clinging to her proper ways. One of the next generation of daughters would lose her husband suddenly, and though nearly in poverty, would still send her three children to college. Well do I know, that one of that woman's daughters, in her time, would lose a daughter and emerge with her faith and self intact. This shortbread is my link to them all. I would wish their wisdom and strength upon me.
Sarah Thorne Mentock

KISIEL (CRANBERRY DESSERT)

This Polish dessert is a tradition at the table of my friend, Marysia, which she shares with us. *Kisiel* is smooth, tart, and delicious as a pudding, or topping for other treats. Serves 6.

1 lb. bag fresh cranberries
Water, to cover cranberries
½ cup sugar or ¼ cup agave, or to taste
Juice of ½ lemon, or to taste
3-4 teaspoons cornstarch
¼ cup additional water

Cover cranberries with water, in a medium pot, bring to boil. Cook until cranberries begin to soften and burst. In a strainer, pour off water, place in a food mill or blender, puree cranberries, place in a bowl with ¼ cup water. Stir in sugar, lemon juice, and cornstarch. Taste for desired sweetness. Consistency should be similar to a thickened soup. Let stand in refrigerator for 1 hour.

Nightshade free
Gluten free
Lactose free

SUMMER PUDDING - A FAVORITE IN THE UK

I was first introduced to Summer Pudding by my English friend, Valerie. Then my friend, Pat, discovered this famous dish while living in London for several years. It truly is an amazing summer's treat, and both of these fine cooks do it right! Serves 8.

10-12 slices white bread
Butter
2 quarts mix of fresh raspberries, blackberries, blueberries, and gooseberries, rinsed well and drained
1 ¼ cups very fine sugar (or ¾ cup agave, or to taste)
Whipping cream, prepared when ready to serve

Remove crusts from bread, cut into triangles, lightly butter bread. Completely line, from top to bottom, a 2 quart deep bowl, or English pudding bowl, overlapping pieces of bread. Save enough bread to cover top. Place fruit in mixing bowl, add sugar and mix well. Gently simmer fruit 4-5 minutes with 1/2 cup water, cool slightly. Ladle fruit mixture into the bread mold, completely cover top with remaining bread. Place a plate on top of the bowl, with a 3-4 pound weight on top. Placefruit mold in refrigerator overnight or for 12 hours. When ready to serve, place a chilled serving plate upside down over the mold. Grasping plate and mold firmly together, quickly invert. The pudding should easily slide out. Serve with whipped cream, for a delicious and beautiful summer dessert.

Nightshade free
Lactose free (omit whipping cream)

ALMOND TORTES

My friend, Martha, chooses this lovely, nightshade free desert for special guests. The fresh berries add color, and the crisps add crunch. The recipe consists of two steps, which assemble for a grand presentation. Serves 8-10.

FOR CRISPS:
¾ cup finely chopped almonds
½ cup sugar
½ cup butter
1 tablespoon flour
2 tablespoons heavy cream

FOR FILLING:
1 cup chilled heavy cream
2 tablespoons packed brown sugar
¼ teaspoon cinnamon
1 dash nutmeg
½ teaspoon pure bourbon vanilla, or pure vanilla extract
Mix of fresh berries

THE CRISPS: Preheat oven to 375 degrees, with rack on lower shelf. Combine all the "crisp ingredients," in a heavy sauce pan. Heat over medium-low heat until butter and sugar completely dissolve. Set aside to cool for about 15 minutes. Line light-colored baking sheets with parchment paper. (Dark baking sheets will burn crisps.) Drop teaspoons of batter 5-6 inches apart on baking sheets. They meld together, and can be cut with a knife when cooled. Bake until lightly browned, about 8 minutes. Cool on baking sheets, on a rack, for 5 minutes, then transfer crisps to rack to completely cool.

THE FILLING: Beat heavy cream in a chilled bowl with an electric mixer, until soft peaks form. Gradually add sugar, being careful not to over-beat. Fold in cinnamon, nutmeg, and vanilla.

TO ASSEMBLE: Place ½ of the almond crisps on a serving tray. Top with a mounded spoonful of the whipped cream, followed with a few berries. Top with an additional crisp, more whipped cream, then a sprinkle of cinnamon, and a few berries. Note: Crisps are very fragile and break easily. Use broken pieces as additional garnish over fresh fruit or ice cream.

Nightshade free

RHUBARB STRAWBERRY COMPOTE

This delicate and delicious dessert is shared by my friend, Julie, which is nightshade and gluten free. Serves 4.

2 cups rhubarb, chopped
½ cup water
¼ cup sugar
Pinch of salt
1 cup strawberries, halved or quartered
Greek yogurt

Place rhubarb, water, sugar, and salt in a saucepan, over medium-heat. Stir as needed until rhubarb softens and begins to break down. Cook until ingredients reach desired consistency. Remove pot from heat, add strawberries, mixing well. Transfer to a container and refrigerate, to thoroughly cool. Serve over Greek yogurt.

Nightshade free
Gluten free

BEVERAGES, SAUCES, AND OTHER FUN STUFF

BEVERAGES, SAUCES, AND OTHER FUN STUFF

To pay homage to *Preserved Lemons* that I use in numerous recipes throughout this book, I begin this section with the following recipe. These lemons are versatile beyond belief, and if you're a lemon aficionado, as I am, you will want to have these on hand year-round.

PRESERVED LEMONS

10-11 whole lemons, washed well
2/3 cup Kosher salt or sea salt
¾ cup olive oil
Bottled lemon juice, as option

Blanche lemons in boiling water for 5 minutes. Drain, cool, cut each lemon into 4 wedges. Discard seeds. Toss in a large bowl with salt and olive oil. Pack into clean jars with lids. (Use 5-7 small jars for easy storage, which also helps to keep lemons fresh.) Squeeze enough juice from extra lemons to cover (or top with bottled lemon juice). Secure lids. Place lemons on kitchen counter at room temperature for 5 days, shaking each day several times, to stir the liquid, or invert for a couple hours each day. At end of 5 days, refrigerate. Lemons will keep for several months. Preserved lemons add pizzazz to fish, chicken, salads, salad dressings, bean and vegetarian dishes, soups/stews, Moroccan and other ethnic cuisines. Preserved lemons make lovely hostess gifts, as well.

Nightshade free
Gluten free
Lactose free

RUBY RED MARY

Few beverages are compromised by nightshades, but one of my all-time favorites, the *Bloody Mary*, became off limits early on as I began my journey with nightshades. However, the following recipe replaces this famed beverage. I hope you'll try this interesting alternative. Serves 1.

In a 10 ounce glass (one serving):
add ice
1-2 ounces of vodka
Ruby Red grapefruit juice, filled to top
Add:
1 squirt fresh lemon juice
White and black peppers, to taste
Worcestershire sauce, to taste
(without chili extract)
½ - 1 teaspoon horseradish
Dash celery salt
Celery stalk, garnish

This beverage can be as spicy as you wish, by adding additional white pepper. Mix ingredients well, garnish with a celery stalk. Please note: Some Worcestershire sauces contain chili extract, which should be avoided for those who are sensitive to nightshades. See recipe for *Prune Enhanced Worcestershire Sauce,* that follows.

Nightshade free
Gluten free
Lactose free

CHRISTMAS CHAMPAGNE WITH POMEGRANATE

For the holidays, try this champagne drink, sparkling with pomegranate arils, the juice sacs from the plant. It's simple, beautiful, and festive around the Christmas tree. Serves 6.

6 champagne flutes
Pomegranate arils

In advance, halve a pomegranate, remove arils from inside the husks. When ready to serve, fill flutes with champagne, add 1 tablespoon arils to each glass.

Nightshade free
Gluten free
Lactose free

GARDENER'S WATER

My gardening friend, Niki, shared this recipe a few years back, which remains a must during the summer months. It is a lifesaver on hot days.

1 quart water
Spritz of lime or lemon juice
1 sprig of basil
1 sprig of mint

Mix in a large pitcher, let stand 1 hour. Refrigerate.

Nightshade free
Gluten free
Lactose free

CAROLINE'S SMOOTHIE

This drink makes a perfect breakfast or quick lunch and is full of protein and flavor. The smoothie, when prepared thick, is similar to ice cream or sorbet. If you want the smoothie texture to be thinner increase the milk and omit yogurt. Other frozen fruits such as blueberries, cherries, peaches, etc. are options for this drink as well. Note: As bananas ripen, peel and place in a large freezer bag for later use in smoothies or banana nut bread.

Serves 1.

IN A BLENDER, PROCESS UNTIL SMOOTH:
1 banana (if frozen, break into pieces)
6-8 strawberries, frozen
1 cup 1 % milk (more, as needed)
½ cup plain low fat Greek yogurt
1 rounded scoop protein powder
(optional, but recommended following surgery or serious illness)
1 -2 tablespoons agave, if desired (or honey)
½ cup bran cereal (optional)

Nightshade free
Gluten free (omit cereal)

PRUNE ENHANCED WORCESTERSHIRE SAUCE

Unfortunately, I have not found a commercial Worcestershire sauce without chili extract that has the same rich, full flavor of original types. However, I developed this sauce that I believe is as good as the original sauces, and it's nightshade free. This version has the thickness and enhanced flavor that is missing in sauces that do not contain chili extract. It's very simple to make as well.

12 oz. commercial Worcestershire Sauce
(without chili extract)
4 prunes, chopped

Place Worcestershire and prunes in a small sauce pan, bring to a boil. Cook 2-3 minutes. Remove from heat, and let stand covered for 2-3 hours. Process to a smooth, luscious texture. Keep refrigerated. If you choose, you can thin this recipe with additional commercial Worcestershire sauce. However, this version is a rich condiment for meats and other uses.

Nightshade, gluten, and lactose free

PEPPERCORN HORSERADISH SAUCE

My daughter, Kelli, inspired the following condiment recipe when she described a commercial sauce her family enjoys with beef, chicken, pork, or fish. This sauce dresses-up something hot off the grill, and is a luscious condiment for sandwiches and burgers of all kinds. You may want to double this recipe. Peppercorns and horseradish provide *heat* for the sauce, but without the harm of nightshades.

½ cup mayonnaise
1 tablespoon Dijon mustard
2-4 tablespoons, horseradish, to taste
1 tablespoon black peppercorn (crushed)

As preferred, peppercorns can be crushed in a mortar and pestle or minced in a small processor. Mix ingredients well. Chill for at least 3 hours before serving.

Nightshade free
Gluten free
Lactose free

HOLIDAY CRANBERRY SAUCE WITH KICK

Here's something red and tangy for the palate. This sauce is a wonderful addition to the holiday table, but also is delicious drizzled over poached pears as a dessert. Layer sauce over cream cheese or goat cheese as a colorful appetizer for a cocktail buffet. Serves 6-8.

12 oz. fresh cranberries, rinsed and drained
1 cup water
1/2 cup agave, or to taste
1 cinnamon stick
2 -3 tablespoons fresh ginger, minced

Combine all ingredients in a small sauce pan, with lid. Heat to bubbling, partially covered to prevent splatters or possible burns. When the cranberries

begin to pop and thicken, stir well, set aside to cool. Serve room temperature or cold. Keeps for several days.
Nightshade free
Gluten free
Lactose free

JEZEBEL SAUCE

This is an unusual sauce for roast pork or turkey, and is luscious over a block of cream cheese, as an appetizer. It's a wonderful condiment for meats, cheeses, or fried egg sandwiches, and another lovely hostess gift.
Makes approximately 5 cups.

1 18 oz. jar apple jelly
1 18 oz. jar pineapple preserves
1 4 oz. horseradish
1 can (2 oz.) dry mustard (4-5 tablespoons), or to taste

Combine apple jelly, pineapple preserves, and horseradish, until smooth. Add dry mustard, to taste. The more mustard you use, the spicier the sauce. Whisk to remove lumps. Place in 4-5 clean jars with lids, and refrigerate overnight. Stores well in freezer (in plastic containers), but will never completely freeze.
Nightshade free
Gluten free
Lactose free

BEST EVER BLUEBERRY SAUCE

When blueberries are in season, take the opportunity to enjoy this delicious sauce, my friend, Jeanne, shared several years ago. I've modified it, using agave in place of sugar. Makes 4 ½ cups. This sauce is a treasure!

2 ¼ cups blueberries and ¼ cup water
¼ cup agave, or to taste (or honey)

½ teaspoon cinnamon
½ teaspoon nutmeg
¼ teaspoon ground cloves
2 tablespoons balsamic vinegar

Mix all ingredients in a sauce pan and simmer for 20 minutes, stirring occasionally. Serve hot or cold, over poached pears, pound cake, or ice cream.

Nightshade free
Lactose free

ROSEMARY AND GARLIC OLIVE OIL

My friend, Cynthia, creates this rich, fragrant olive oil, which is a delightful gift during the holidays. This olive oil has numerous uses and never fails to please. Try in salad dressings, as a dip with crusty Italian breads, or in marinades.

Quart of olive oil
5-6 sprigs fresh rosemary
6-8 garlic cloves, crushed

Place rosemary and crushed garlic cloves in a decorative bottle, add olive oil to top of container. Tightly close. This oil keeps at room temperature for a couple weeks, but should be refrigerated later. When ready to use chilled oil, set out for 30 minutes, prior to use. Makes 1 quart.

Nightshade free
Gluten free
Lactose free

CAROLINE'S DRY SPICY RUB

This rub is a spicy alternative to marinades and can be used with chicken, meats, and firm fish. Combine ingredients below, place in a small food processor. Process until finely ground. When ready to use, press rub into flesh of foods you are preparing to grill or roast. After applying rub, refrigerate meats/fish for several hours. To increase flavors, use additional rub and refrigerate longer. Make extra rub and store in a tightly closed container. Note: To add crispness to foods, after rub is applied and just before cooking, lightly drizzle olive oil over items to be roasted or grilled. If you choose, this rub can be used as a marinade by adding olive oil with fresh lemon or lime juice.

DRY SPICY RUB

1 tablespoon coarse black pepper

1 tablespoon Kosher salt

1 teaspoon garlic flakes

1 teaspoon onion powder or dried onion flakes

1 tablespoon Italian herb mix (or dried oregano)

1 tablespoon black peppercorn

1-2 teaspoon white pepper (more for extra heat)

1 teaspoon turmeric

1 teaspoon dry mustard

Nightshade free

Gluten free

Lactose free

SALSA VERDE

If you have a sensitivity to nightshades, but love tangy foods, you may be missing salsas. My friend, Dasha, shares this Argentinean relish that is perfect for beef, chicken, and firm fish. The original recipe is from *Two Dudes, One Pan.* Serves 2-3 with entrée.

1/3 cup olive oil

Juice and zest of 1 lemon

2 anchovy fillets, finely minced

2 garlic cloves, finely minced

1 tablespoon capers, roughly chopped
1 tablespoon fresh oregano, chopped
1 tablespoon flat leaf parsley, chopped
1 teaspoon mint, finely chopped
1/2 teaspoon Kosher salt

Blend ingredients well, serve room temperature.

Nightshade free
Gluten free
Lactose free

THREE ROASTING-TOASTING TREATS ...... TO HAVE ON HAND

Some Saturday afternoon, take an hour or so, to prepare **roasted garlic, toasted oats, and toasted walnuts.** These are fun to prepare, and store easily in the pantry or freezer. When a recipe calls for one of these special additions, you'll be ready. They are nightshade, gluten, and lactose free. Although, research on oats, indicates that this grain may contain limited gluten.

ROASTED GARLIC

Preheat oven to 375 degrees. Line a cookie sheet with foil coated with vegetable oil spray. Spread 2-3 cups peeled garlic cloves over the foil (available in bulk at many supermarkets), then place in oven for 40-45 minutes or until garlic becomes fragrant and the skin glistens and lightly browns. Be careful not to burn. Set aside, to cool. Store in freezer bags.

USES: When a recipe calls for garlic, try this roasted version instead of raw garlic. The enhanced flavor is a pleasant surprise. Roasted garlic mashes easily in mayonnaise to create a simple condiment or garlic aioli.

ROASTED WALNUTS (or other nuts)

Preheat oven to 300 degrees, place walnuts in a single layer on a dry, foil liner on a cookie sheet. Roast 10-15 minutes, or until slightly golden and fragrant. Be careful not to burn.

USES: When walnuts are roasted, the flavor explodes. These crunchy nuts add punch to almost anything, such as salads, pastas, and is the perfect healthy snack.

TOASTED OATS

Preheat oven to 350 degrees. Evenly spread 4-6 cups of oats in a dry shallow baking pan. Place in oven, using a timer in 15 minute intervals to check progress and to stir. Roasting oats in the oven, depending on amount, can take 20-30 minutes. Be careful not to burn. Roast until golden brown and the oats become fragrant. Cool thoroughly. Store in large sealed plastic bags or container, with lid.

USES: Oatmeal is the main-stay of breakfasts around the country everyday of the week. However, toasted oats become a special breakfast when served with berries, banana, yogurt, and a touch of agave. Toasted oats are also a lovely garnish for salads, soups, sandwiches, etc. Mix with toasted nuts and dried fruits, for a nutty flavored snack.

Nightshade free
Gluten free
Lactose free

MISO GLAZE

This glaze, offered by my friend, Marysia, provides a beautiful and delicious finish for fish. This recipe makes a large batch, and keeps well in the refrigerator for several months.

8 oz. white miso paste

½ bottle Mirin cooking wine, or to taste

1 cup sugar, or to taste

In a double-boiler, add miso paste, slowly blend in wine. As miso begins to melt, carefully whisk the sugar into mixture. When very smooth and golden, cool. Refrigerate in tightly closed container. **For use on fish:** Grill, roast, or broil as desired, when done, brush or spoon glaze over fish. Place under hot broiler for 1 minute. Glaze will have a rich, golden color and brown spots that look like it is beginning to burn. Remove immediately and serve.

Nightshade free

Gluten free

Lactose free

EPILOGUE

Another side of my personal story

My primary focus throughout this book has been on nightshade plants and the harm they cause some individuals suffering with arthritis. This focus has also included emphasis on gluten and lactose intolerance. However as I conclude, I want to share a side of my personal story that may be of help to others. Since writing the cookbook, and because of my passion for food and creating recipes, it's important to me to give full disclosure because with passion, comes responsibility.

After many years of struggling with my weight, diets, and poor self-image, I discovered that I have an eating disorder. Like so many people with eating disorders, my problem began in early childhood. My issue takes the form of excessive eating, in particular, the uncontrollable eating of foods with sugar and chocolate. Like an alcoholic with that first drink, when I took the first bite, there was no stopping.

I have been on a diet of some kind my entire life, beginning at the age of thirteen. I weighed myself the moment my feet hit the floor each morning and followed my first weigh-in of the day with numerous weigh-ins throughout the day. I was never happy with my weight, even when I was very thin, and I *never* started a diet without planning how to reward myself when I reached my goal weight. There was only one plan and it was always the same: I would eat all the chocolate my heart desired. However, with that one act, the old eating habits and binges returned, starting the yo-yo diet game once again.

Several years ago I discovered a 12-Step Program called Overeaters Anonymous (OA). This program, its principles, and tools for living a sane life around food dramatically changed me. These principles gave me a way to clarify and maintain portion control and eliminate foods that trigger my binges, such as chocolate and sugar. It's a lifelong path for me and without OA, my weight would still be up and down ten to fifteen pounds every year.

I'm often asked if I feel deprived living without nightshades, and especially living without sugar and chocolate. The answer is simple. Nightshades cause me severe arthritis pain and inflammation, so why would I eat foods that make me suffer? In the same regard, being over-weight has caused mental and physical anguish my entire life, so why would I want to suffer in that way? Freedom from any pain is a precious gift.

The obesity problem in the United States is serious. It affects us all, and it's dangerous on many levels. I know as well as anyone how difficult it is to maintain a reasonable weight and to eat responsibly, but it's important. It's important for us as adults, but also for our children and grandchildren, whom we influence. The obesity epidemic affects arthritis and joint deterioration, heart disease, cancer, diabetes, and blood pressure. What are we doing to ourselves and to our children? The long-term effects are often permanent, frightening, and fatal.

Therefore, when I talk about my passion for cooking and enjoying good food, I need to add that I also have a passion for being responsible with food. In the beginning, it was difficult to give up nightshade foods, which I truly loved. It was also difficult to give up sugar and chocolate. Neither is difficult any longer, because I don't go there. I can't. Most importantly, the elimination of these foods has given me a richer, healthier, and saner life. No, I don't feel deprived. I'm grateful. Grateful that I know about the effects of nightshades and how they impact my arthritis and grateful that I came to grips with my eating disorder.

Be well and blessed with peace.

The greatest power on earth is the power of a made-up mind.
Les Brown, inspirational speaker, Memphis, Tennessee

CAROLINE THOMPSON

Life Bio

I am a daughter, sister, wife, mother, stepmother, grandmother of eight, niece, aunt, and friend. I take these roles seriously and do my best to do them well. Thankfully, my life has been rich and full.

My professional life in business development began when I was twenty-one years of age at a small country bank in southeast Missouri. The position included hosting a local radio show each week called *The Lady from the Bank.* After moving to Memphis, Tennessee, the big city in my region, my banking career led to fundraising and institutional advancement for the University of Memphis, and later as the executive director of the Baptist Medical Center Foundation, in Oklahoma City, Oklahoma. While in Oklahoma City, I met and married George Thompson, who is still my best friend and continues to support my wildest dreams, such as writing this cookbook.

When I discovered the world of painting and art, George was there to cheer me on. My adventures into art emerged as a central focus for me in 2000, leading to a rewarding career. However, throughout my life cooking, creating recipes, and entertaining have been sources of delight and artistic outlets.

Fourteen years ago, I suddenly and unexpectedly developed arthritis in my hands. This disease, and its effect on my overall health, dramatically changed the recipes I traditionally cooked and the foods I enjoyed eating.

Because a friend spoke up and told me about nightshade plants and their effect on arthritis, I discovered that these types of vegetables compromise and inflame my type of arthritis. I quickly began to develop recipes and foods that I could safely eat but thoroughly enjoy. The collection of recipes in *Caroline's No Nightshade Kitchen: Arthritis Diet* are either original or have been modified to be nightshade free. Several friends, who are excellent cooks, have provided nightshade free recipes for your enjoyment. Many of the recipes are also gluten and lactose free. This book has given me the opportunity to share my love of cooking, my recipes, and the phenomenon associated with nightshade plants.

Over many years, my interest in cooking and fine foods has been enriched through participation in numerous cooking classes and workshops. Instruction has included Italian, French, and Cajun cuisines; pastry and desserts; as well as many other specialty foods. These classes provided luscious foods to enhance my table as well as inspiration for original creations.

In the late 1990s, I completed an intensive French cooking course at the Cooking School of the Rockies in Boulder, Colorado. This four-month-long course included instruction for basic French cuisine, such as classic vinaigrette, quiche, sauces, fish and meats, and specialty techniques such as flambé.

In 1997, I completed a twelve-day workshop at the Institut Paul Bocuse in Lyon, France. My study there featured instruction in French regional cuisine, wine selection, cheese, pastry techniques, and French cooking terminology. The workshop included field study at local fish, meat, chocolate, and vegetable markets.

Cooking remains a joy in my life, as does eating a diet that is healthy, rich in flavor, and free of nightshade vegetables.

APPENDIX

RELATED RESOURCES

ORGANIZATIONS:

Arthritis Nightshades Research Foundation
3906 N.W. 31st Place
Gainesville, Fl 32606
www.noarthritis.com/foundation

BOOKS:

Balch, Phyllis A., C.N.C. ***Prescription for Nutritional Healing***, Penguin Group, USA, 2010
"Consumption of certain plants, called nightshades, may worsen arthritis symptoms"

Childers, Dr. Norman. ***Arthritis-Childers' Diet That Stops It!*** Childers Publications, 1999.
Includes case histories with comments based on over 1400 cooperators on the no-nightshades diet for 1-20 years.

Claudio, Patricia, and Vogel, Joan. ***Arthritis-Free Cooking,*** Norman Childers Publications, 1999.
"There are no Nightshades in this cookbook!"

Fowler, Michael. ***Nightshade Free Pain Free!*** Grass Fire Media, 2007.

Rogers, Sherry A, M.D., ***Pain free in Six Weeks***, Prestige Publishing, 2001
Dr. Rogers advises a three-month trial of the no-nightshades diet for anyone in chronic arthritis pain.

PUBLISHED RESEARCH PAPER:

N.F. Childers, Ph.D. and M.S. Margoles, M.D., "An Apparent Relation of Nightshades (Solanaceae) to Arthritis." *Journal of Neurological and Orthopedic Medical Surgery* (1993) 12:227-231.
"Diet appears to be a factor in the etiology of arthritis based on surveys of over 1400 volunteers during a 20-year period. Plants in the drug family, *Solanaceae* (nightshades) are an important causative factor in arthritis in sensitive people."

NIGHTSHADES TOXICITY INFORMATION:

http://doctorklaper.com/answers07.html
DoctorKlaper.com- Official Website for Dr. Michael Klaper,
Diet, Arthritis, and Autoimmune Diseases, "The Most Likely Culprits", by Dr. Klaper, 2011

http://www.pcrm.org/health/health-topics/foods-and-arthritis
Physicians Committee For Responsible Medicine,
Foods and Arthritis – The Four Week Anti-Arthritis Diet

http://macrobiotics.co.uk/articles/nightshades.htm
Macrobiotic Guide,
Nightshades, by Norman F. Childers, PhD,

http://www.sciencedirect.com/science/article/pii/0049017291900522

Science Direct,

Seminars in Arthritis and Rheumatism, Vol. 21, Issue 1, August 1991, Pg. 12-23

Rheumatoid Arthritis, Food, and Allergy, by M.A.F.J. van de Laar, MD, PhD (Rheumatologist), J.K. van der Korst, MD. PhD (Professor of Rheumatology)

www.naturalnews.com/027978_nightshade_vegetables.html

Natural News,

Nightshade Vegetables may Cause Adverse Reactions in Some People, Deanne Dean, January, 2010.

http://www.realfooduniversity.com/nightshades/

Real Food University,

Do Nightshades Promote Inflammation? By Scott Kustes

http://www.arthritisresearchuk.org/arthritis-information/arthritis-and-daily-life/diet-and-arthritis/should-i-avoid-certain-foods.aspx

Arthritis Research UK,

Arthritis Information: Should I Avoid Certain Foods?

http://www.getting-started-with-healthy-eating.com/no-nightshades-diet.html

getting-started-with-healthy-eating.com,

How to do a No Nightshades Diet, by Heidi Boudro, 2012

http://www.livestrong.com/article/436546-nightshade-vegetables-arthritis/

Livestrong.com,

Nightshade Vegetables and Arthritis by Cindi Eli, July 17, 2011

Nightshade Vegetables and Rheumatoid Arthritis, January 19, 2011

http://rxalternativemedicine.com/blog/index.php/category/arthritis/
Rx Alternative Medicine,
Arthritis Alternative Medicine by Dr. James Smith, May 2, 2011

http://whfoods.com/genpage.php?tname=george&dbid=62
The World's Healthiest Foods,
What are Nightshades and in Which Foods Are They Found?
The George Mateljan Foundation

http://www.diagnose-me.com/treat/T427498.html
Diagnose-me.com,
Nightshade Family Food Avoidance, January 22, 2012

INDEX

B

C

D

E

F

G

T

V

W

Z

CPSIA information can be obtained
at www.ICGtesting.com
Printed in the USA
BVHW061920181220
595947BV00009B/491